Autistic Spectr ~~

14 DAY BOOK

East Riding College ~ Learning Resour~

Please return this item on or before the last date stamped below.

~~ ~~ ~~ before the due date -

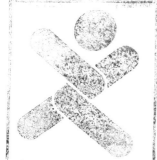

Autistic Spectrum Disorders in the Secondary School

Lynn Plimley
Maggie Bowen

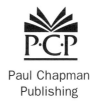

Paul Chapman
Publishing

Paul Chapman Publishing
A SAGE Publications Company
1 Oliver's Yard
55 City Road
London EC1Y 1SP

SAGE Publications Inc
2455 Teller Road
Thousand Oaks, California 91320

SAGE Publications India Pvt Ltd
B-42, Panchsheel Enclave
Post Box 4109
New Delhi 110 017

Library of Congress Control Number 2006920090

A catalogue record for this book is available from the
British Library

ISBN-10 1-4129-2310-7   ISBN-13 978-1-4129-2310-1
ISBN-10 1-4129-2311-5   ISBN-13 978-1-4129-2311-8 (pbk)

Typeset by C&M Digitals (P) Ltd., Chennai, India
Printed in Great Britain by the Cromwell Press, Trowbridge, Wiltshire
Printed on paper from sustainable resources

Contents

Acknowledgements		viii
How to use this book		ix
1	Making good transitions from primary school	1
2	Considering the environment	7
3	Inclusive practice and whole-school approaches	16
4	Planning the curriculum for access and accreditation	22
5	Social strategies: helping pupils to cope	27
6	Observation and recording	34
7	Working with sensory differences	40
8	Preparing for work experience and future employment	48
9	Adolescence, sexuality and PSHE	53
10	Developing partnerships with parents	59
11	Managing challenging behaviour	64
12	Issues relating to mental health and the criminal justice system	70
13	Educating colleagues	76
References		80
Glossary		83
Index		85

Lynn Plimley

Lynn Plimley originally trained to teach children with Special Educational Needs in the mid-70s, and since 1979 has worked with children with autistic spectrum disorders (ASD). She has worked in generic special schools for primary aged children, residential schools for those with SLD and been part of a multi-disciplinary team supporting inclusion. She was the first Principal of Coddington Court School in Herefordshire, a provision for children aged 8–19 with ASD.

She works part-time as a Lecturer in ASD at the University of Birmingham on their web-based course (www.webautism.bham.ac.uk). She also tutors M.Ed dissertation students for the Course in ASD (Distance Learning), and is a member of the internationally respected Autism team, based at the University of Birmingham's School of Education, led by Professor Rita Jordan.

Lynn also works for Autism Cymru, establishing a mechanism for main-stream Secondary, Primary and Special school teachers, to share good practice. She offers consultancy as a trainer for any kind of provision for people with ASD, and has built up a national profile of training in the importance of understanding the condition of autistic spectrum disorders for schools and care establishments. Lynn is the Book Editor, and an Editorial Board member, of the *Good Autism Practice Journal*.

Maggie Bowen

Maggie gained her academic and professional qualifications at universities in Aberystwyth, Leeds and Bangor. She began her teaching career in a school for children with severe learning difficulties (SLD), and went on to work as a Community Liaison Teacher for individuals with SLD. She has been a Team Inspector of secondary and special schools and a Threshold Assessor, and has worked as part of a multi-agency team responsible for developing a range of new services for individuals of all ages with Severe Learning Difficulties (SLD).

She was Programme Leader for Special Educational Needs courses and the MA in Education at the North East Wales Institute of Higher Education (NEWI). She has worked for the Welsh Assembly Government as Development Officer for Inclusion in Wales with a specific responsibility for Autistic Spectrum Disorders (ASD), Able and Talented and SEN Training in Wales.

She joined the team at Autism Cymru as Head of Public and Voluntary Sector Partnerships/Deputy CEO in January 2005. She has published on a range of SEN issues in books and journals, and is still committed to training and consultancy work with a range of practitioners from health, social services, education, the criminal justice system and the emergency services.

Acknowledgements

Our sincere thanks go to a range of people who have helped us gather evidence for this book, in particular members of the Autism Cymru Secondary School Forum, Dr Verity Donnelly, Dr Patrick Loughran, SNAP Cymru, Play Radnor, Ray Dickson, Jude Bowen and NoMAD.

How to use this book

This book has been designed as a resource that readers will want to dip into when they are working with pupils with ASD in the secondary school or secondary special school. Many examples are given that address issues arising from setting up specific bases or resources within the secondary school, but the authors also recognise that these ideas and strategies can be used in whole school planning. The authors have drawn upon the current state of knowledge and legislation and the good practice of many secondary school teachers to cover issues and strategies that are not necessarily available elsewhere.

The book assumes a working knowledge and understanding of the condition of ASD and covers in further depth the impact of sensory differences. Practical ideas and strategies are given to address typical secondary school issues, and key times during the pupil's life in a secondary school, adolescence and their routes post school are dealt with.

The authors know from their strong links with secondary school teachers that many of the chapters deal with situations and issues that can occur from time to time in their work with pupils with ASD. They hope that this resource goes some way to expanding on information and knowledge that is currently available.

Making good transitions
from primary school

This chapter examines issues around transition planning and the need to involve a wide range of personnel in the process. It suggests a range of strategies that may be used to gradually introduce the new environment.

With current educational trends moving towards more mainstream inclusion for children on the autistic spectrum (DfES, 2001; WAG, 2003; Audit Scotland/HMIe 2003), the sooner the familiarization exercises start with the new environment and population, the better. Parents who have chosen mainstream primary schools for their youngsters with ASD can often feel unsettled when they are looking at secondary provision. Some might be concerned that the secondary environment is too large and too busy for their child and may even consider a special-school placement. In some instances local education authorities may have developed ASD resource bases attached to a designated mainstream school. In such instances, transition planning between primary and secondary phases should be easier.

Table 1.1 illustrates some of the common differences between educational provision.

With greater emphasis on league tables and Standardized Assessment Tasks (SATs) in some parts of the UK, larger primary schools may be moving towards a similar model of provision and support as secondary schools. However, the difference between the two environments which may not suit the child with ASD is the sense of *local* provision at primary, i.e. most are located within the child's community, parents know staff and vice versa.

Table 1.1   Common differences between types of schools

Mainstream		
Primary	**Secondary**	**Special**
Child-centred	Microcosm of society	Everyone is equal
Friendly ethos	Efficient ethos	Understanding ethos
Local	Travel may be needed	Travel with transport
Local friendships	Local/distance friends	Friends hard to sustain
One teacher for all subjects	One teacher per subject	Mix of two
Good parent links	Parents' evenings	Good parental contact
Curriculum differentiated	Subject streaming	Individualized curriculum
Parent support informal	Parent contact formal	High pupil/staff ratios
Extra help/tuition on site	Extra help is external	

A secondary school may be at a distance from home and only accessible on school transport. The lack of personal contact and the efficient ethos of secondary schools, with a high emphasis on conformity, may mean that mainstream in Year 7 is a very difficult option for parents and carers to accept.

However, with careful planning many obstacles can be overcome. For example, more inclusive secondary schools are taking greater responsibility when it comes to easing the transition of pupils with disabilities by early and effective exercises to support their future learners. Proactive secondary special educational needs coordinators (SENCos) are in touch with their primary counterparts and will be in a dialogue with their feeder primary schools to identify pupils in need of support by as early as Year 4 or 5. This may make all the difference to transition across phases being a success. It is quite common if the child has had a proportion of 1:1 support in the primary school for that to continue into the secondary provision but not by the same person. Support contracts are issued and attached to a certain number of hours for a named child within a particular setting and this may terminate once the child moves to a new setting. Often a new member of support staff will be appointed with a different contract. Although this is understandable, it can be another change that the child has to learn to accept and therefore needs careful consideration in transition planning.

We offer the following suggestions for successful transition planning:

- Procedures outlined in the SEN Code of Practice (WAG, 2001/DfES, 2002b) should be noted
- The views, feelings and anxieties of the child with ASD should be considered at all times
- Secondary and primary SENCos have regular dialogue throughout the school year

- Secondary SENCo attends annual reviews of children with a Statement of Special Need in Year 5 and Year 6
- Child with an ASD visits the secondary school as often as possible in the summer term, prior to the open day when all potential Year 7 students attend
- Nominated member of secondary staff gives pastoral support to the child early on
- There should be adequate record-keeping and profiling methods so that all relevant information can accompany individuals with ASD as they move on.
- Parents of child with ASD are invited into secondary school to talk about their child's differences
- Staff make up an action plan around the support needs of the child
- Sensory and environmental adjustments are pre-empted and accommodated
- The secondary environment is labelled and made more visually clear
- The secondary environment is made into a CD-ROM 'virtual map' as a guide for all new pupils (Cook and Stowe, 2003) well in advance of their start date
- All secondary staff have awareness-raising session using cases studies of pupils with ASD that they know
- The secondary environment has a breaktime "safe haven" room available for all vulnerable pupils
- The secondary SENCo has a portable file of accessible information on all conditions present in the pupil population of the school
- The secondary SENCo has quick checklists for each teacher containing guidance on how to teach pupils with different conditions
- There is a peer buddy system in place
- There is a 'circle of friends' (Whitaker, Barratt, Joy, Potter and Thomas, 1998) mechanism within school
- All channels for communication are kept open

CASE STUDY

Background to setting up a secondary base

Work began on the concept of setting up a secondary school base in 1996, as more and more pupils coming into Year 7 had a diagnosis of ASD. The principal educational psychologist in our LEA had

(Continued)

(Continued)

studied ASD in some depth and she managed to convince her SEN colleagues at County Hall that a base would be a good provision to set up to help to ease the transition of pupils with ASD. It was seen as a natural progression that the pupils in the primary bases for ASD would feed into a secondary base. We were given a Portakabin in the school yard and a specialist teacher, Jim, was appointed as Teacher in Charge a term before our new pupils began in September. Jim spent his first term visiting prospective pupils at their schools/ at home and appointing three teaching assistants (TAs) to work 1:1 with the proposed intake of four pupils with ASD. He also worked hard with the principal educational psychologist on running awareness-raising for all of the school's staff (secretaries and lunchtime supervisors included). He invited other teachers working with children with ASD to run workshops and set up an 'interest group' where school staff and parents could meet once a month to discuss important issues.

All of the forward planning and preparation paid off in the Autumn Term and there were very few teething problems. However, what had not been apparent before opening the base was that there was a wide range of ability level in the first intake of four students. They all had a diagnosis of ASD, but the actual range of their level of ability varied enormously. What was also highly variable was each individual's patchy functioning in any one particular subject or in communication and social interaction. The staff team in the base decided that they needed to spend time observing each individual and then to work together to find imaginative solutions. It became apparent that all of the staff within the base needed to look beyond academic subjects and focus on an holistic view of each child.

Training role of the staff at the base

By doing the preparation and training of the school's staff, Jim and his TAs found that they had had an impact upon:

- How subject teachers delivered their lessons, what learning styles they were catering for and where there were gaps

(Continued)

- How the language of instruction was delivered, with emphasis on use of minimal language, the child's name prefacing the instruction ('Tom, I want you to go through this passage and underline...') and the back-up of some visual reference so that the child was encouraged to be as independent as possible
- How the classroom environment was arranged, where the child sat, the use of good peer role models for pair work
- The whole staff looked at enhancing the range of accredited courses at 14–16 to include 'Entry Level' qualifications in all subjects alongside GCSEs.

Getting to know each child as an individual

The staff in the Base forged strong relationships with each of the pupils. They took time to learn from the child's family – they, after all, are the experts in their child/brother/sister. They thought of the functional skills and abilities each child would need as they got older and instigated social skills training, use of leisure facilities, community skills and personal care skills including sex education. As these Base children moved up through the school, they needed less support from the Base staff and they were more included in the life of the school. However, each child retained a soft spot for the base staff and used their facilities at times when the demands of school life became too much for them. Jim and his staff were happy to provide a 'safe haven' for these students and their needs continued to be catered for within the Base.

From an original case study by Christine Hickman, University of Northampton

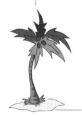

REFLECTIVE OASIS

How would you organize staff to build relationships with new pupils?

How would you gain important information from parents and families?

Points to remember

- Plan for transition early
- Involve a range of personnel, parents and pupils
- Consider a range of strategies to introduce the new environment

2

Considering the environment

This chapter emphasises the importance of creating an ASD-friendly environment and focuses on whole-school issues, classroom issues, sensory considerations and health and safety.

Whole-school issues

The 'Good Practice Guidance' (DfES, 2002a) for schools in England includes pointers that examine where LEAs and schools can influence the success of inclusion for pupils with ASD. These include:

- Policies and procedures to support those with ASD
- Availability of training and INSET for staff at all levels
- Staff awareness
- Accessibility of pupil information
- Workable strategies and interventions
- Empathy and support mechanisms for the individual
- Good preparation for transitions

The authors of the Good Practice pointers are aware that a lot of the suggestions will only be achieved over time and only with the goodwill and strong motivation of all concerned.

Although the guidance pertains to schools within England, Scotland and Wales have used this model and impetus to create their own framework. Also these pointers were written specifically with the provision for children with ASD in mind, but they have validity in the area of adult services too.

The concept of autism-friendliness in design

For a number of years those designing new, or adapting old, environments for children and adults with ASD have pondered over decisions concerning paint colours, types of lighting, types of heating, use of natural light, and construction of basic resources/facilities. There is very little written about the topic.

In order to design for people with ASD, there is a number of principles that could apply (Plimley, 2004). The primary one is to consult the people for whom it is intended.

New provision

In contemplating where to site a new provision for those with ASD, attention needs to be paid to:

- How close is the local community?
- What is the community view on the provision?
- What are the major routes to the provision like?
- How close are emergency facilities?
- Where will the staffing travel from and what is the local employment market like?

When considering setting up a unit, adapting existing provision or making your school as inclusive as possible, there is good advice from Bishop (2001). As a DfES architect he looked at enabling access and participation in the whole of school life for those children with SEN. He points out three basic principles that can enable a high level of participation:

1. Making sure that all students have access to resources and specialist areas, thereby ensuring access to the whole curriculum.
2. Having a good level of access to the enriched curriculum – dining, drama, play, sport, library and assembly facilities.
3. Focus on the importance of personal welfare and health and safety issues.

Visser (2001) examines the importance of environment, resources, ergonomics and staffing factors for children with emotional and behavioural difficulties (EBD). There appears to be a correlation between poor environment, crumbling and vandalized buildings, poor public areas and lack of a communal school pride in their surroundings with schools that have been rated by Ofsted as being in 'serious difficulties' or 'special measures'. Visser argues that emphasis on making the school look both functional and attractive strongly conveys the expectations of the learning that will take place there.

He suggests that any physical and environmental arrangements must meet the needs of the pupils it is designed for. This is especially true for pupils with ASD. He points to the importance of the following factors when looking at classroom and school organisation:

- Having a space of one's own
- Having space between furniture
- Good storage facilities for equipment, resources and personal possessions
- Looking at ergonomic features of environments – heating, lighting, temperature and acoustics and possibilities for provoking stress
- Using music to maintain calm
- Having any unit provision *within* the school, not on the periphery.

Classroom planning issues

Within the provision we also need to consider:

What types of equipment/furnishings are there?
What are the evident health and safety dangers?
How are these dealt with?
How accessible are toilet and catering facilities?
How is their design enabling pupil independence?

When designing a room for pupils with ASD, there's a sense of freedom to make your own choices. An exercise to canvass the opinions of six Master's level students (studying ASD) discussed what variables were important in making an 'autism-friendly design' (Plimley, 2004). The students focused on human qualities and environmental factors as key elements. Table 2.1 shows their choices.

These are principles that can be applied in all types of setting for individuals with ASD. If you are able to make decisions for a new base/room/provision, then attention will need to be paid to the following choices.

Table 2.1   Human Qualities and Environmental Factors when Working with ASD

Human Qualities	Environmental Factors
Empathetic staff team	Quiet, calm atmosphere
Knowledge of ASD	Carpeted areas
Ability to prioritise the important	Absence of loud, sudden noises
Weighing up issues of conformity	Planning for changes
Consistency and continuity	Visual supports
Personal attitudes towards disability	Adult : child ratios
Evaluating your input	Diffused lighting
Anticipation of what might happen next	Sensory factors - being able to screen, cut out or adapt
	Muted colours
	Paying attention to visual perceptions

Design factors

The following need consideration:

- Room size
- Number of people to be accommodated within the space (including staff)
- Colour and type of wall covering
- Type of flooring and floor covering
- Type of window and safety factors re exit/breakages
- Type of door and ease of access/exit and where doors are placed
- Number of switches/sockets
- Usage of the room for other functions
- Number of lighting points and type of lighting
- Amount of natural light, (think year-round)
- Type of heating
- Fixed furniture items, e.g. cupboards/shelves
- Amount of floor space

Never underestimate the amount of space that will be needed in the room. More will be needed if you intend to demarcate certain areas for certain activities. Do not forget that for every child with ASD there may be an adult, so double the space, and seating will be needed. Storage space can get overlooked – you may need to lock away some tempting items (e.g. computer) or at least have enough storage to be able to be self-sufficient. Having running water and a sink may be useful, although children with ASD can be attracted to taps and sinks. However, having a water supply increases the number of activities you can offer; not just subject-oriented, but also making drinks independently or teaching kitchen skills.

Colour

Some will say that particular colours are a complete non-starter when decorating rooms to be used by people with ASD. With colour, as with so many other things, people with ASD confound us by being predictably unpredictable. It is important to take the wishes and preferences of the individual into consideration and to adopt a neutral stance (and colour scheme) where there are conflicting likes and dislikes among individuals. If they cannot communicate their colour preferences, consult with those who know the child well or analyse which colours they choose in paint/crayons.

Use of dedicated space

If the space within the environment allows for personal space, a table or a chair that can be allocated to each person will enable someone with an ASD to 'know' where to sit or use table-top activities. If your approach is following TEACCH structured teaching ideas (Mesibov, Shea and Schopler, 2004) then being able to provide dedicated work stations or office areas may guide your use of space.

New furniture

The aesthetic attractiveness of uniform height and colour of furniture can be problematic because people are not designed to fit one size of table and chair. A range of different sizes should be provided because even children of the same age differ greatly in height and width. We all differ in our dimensions, especially young people going through adolescence. Make sure that a seated pupil is able to put their back against the chair while also resting both feet on the floor. Provide adjustable footrests under tables for extra comfort.

Other equipment

Within the classroom a range of equipment can be useful (ACCAC, 2000, p. 15):

- Display boards for visual schedules
- Start and finish boxes
- Portable language aids/laptop computers
- Sound beams
- A digital camera
- Individual folders

Space and storage areas will be needed for this equipment.

Lighting

Consider how the room will be lit and go for low-glare surfaces that will not reflect the sunlight or artificial lighting. Aim for a good level of natural light to avoid reliance upon artificial sources. Think carefully about strip lighting – people with ASD say it can overstimulate their senses.

Other ergonomic factors include overall temperature and access to furniture within the space. Think of the level of activity likely within the room and adjust the temperature accordingly. It is a good idea to opt for adjustable heating as conditions vary from activity to activity. Have areas within the room that can be used for different functions, so that expectations are conveyed visually. Use another area for transitions, as recommended by TEACCH (www.teacch.com).

CASE STUDY

Designing an environment from scratch

While we were able to choose all the interior features of our new unit, we were limited by the design of the building. The rooms to be used for teaching were tiny and there was one other large room. Only one of the classrooms had a storeroom/cupboard. We were lucky to have a shower room with toilet plus an additional separate toilet in the building. The architect had worked on the notion of five children in each room plus one adult.

We had five boys with ASD and some challenging behaviour that needed a decent amount of personal space and a staffing ratio of 2 adults:5 children.

The staff made a viable plan:

- The storeroom/cupboard had a window and extractor put into it so that it could be used as a 1:1 room.
- We persuaded the head of the school to 'give' the unit another storeroom, and have it converted for the same use.
- So both class bases had 1:1 withdrawal rooms.
- The large additional room in the unit was designated as a communal meeting room. A high shelf was put up in there running around the entire circumference of the room. Personal possessions (e.g. CD players, Gameboys) could be stored there and used as a reward.

(Continued)

- More storage cupboards, with roll-top fronts and locks, were put into the classrooms.
- High shelves were put in both classrooms.
- Vertical blinds were removed.
- A fence was put up around the outside play area.
- Window glass was strengthened.
- Fluorescent lights were avoided.
- The heating had thermostats that enabled the staff to control it.
- A carpet distinguished between 'work' and 'play' areas.
- Tall furniture was used to partition the room.
- Three individual workstations were created down one side of the room.
- Red tables and chairs were used here.
- Blue tables and chairs were used elsewhere. Children could see the difference between independent work and other activities.

There were constraints in the size of the setting – we had to use the same table for snack time and group work.

In appointing staff, I looked for personal qualities rather than experience. Training can be given, but other qualities and attitudes are essential in this field. People who had an interest in something different to the norm, people who had a 'spark' to their personalities, people with humour, people with qualities or skills that were complementary to the needs of the youngsters in the unit. Another teacher and four TAs (two later to be trained and given new job descriptions as play specialist and music specialist) were appointed.

In the beginning we had a 'no displays' rule. Some children would rip them, enjoying the tactile, sensory effect, which led to a spiral of challenging behaviour and confrontation. Walls were kept plain, apart from where the children's schedules and choice boards were. Once the children settled and developed in terms of their interaction and communication, we began to introduce some displays that were meaningful to the children.

(Continued)

(Continued)

To conclude, the unit drew upon the expertise of carefully chosen staff, who were committed to a common purpose. The emphasis on de-stressing the environment was essential for all those in it.

(With grateful thanks to Christine Hickman, University of Northampton)

REFLECTIVE OASIS

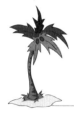

What would be your priorities in setting up something from scratch?

How important would it be to have staff trained in ASD?

Would you go for a TEACCH-inspired environment?

Managing working environments

Schools can be visually stimulating places that place a strong emphasis on social interaction. All teachers, support staff, including midday supervisors and caretaking staff, will need to be sensitive to the needs of pupils with ASD. It is crucial that everyone involved works in a consistent manner. Mixed messages about rules and protocols can be difficult for pupils with ASD to understand when they rely so much on a clear structure to their lives.

We all work best without distraction. For pupils with ASD, it may be necessary to identify a small area of the classroom where they can work independently and with limited 'interference' from other pupils. It is important that pupils with ASD are able to work in a clutter-free environment where resources are clearly labelled. Visual timetables can be very useful in helping pupils to understand the structure of the school day and predict changes. This is especially important in the secondary school where pupils are expected to move around the school for different lessons. Any changes in the room will need careful planning – a pupil with ASD might find it very difficult to do mathematics in a room which by its displays is usually used for geography.

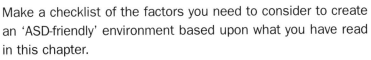

REFLECTIVE OASIS

Make a checklist of the factors you need to consider to create an 'ASD-friendly' environment based upon what you have read in this chapter.

What things do you need to do to make the school environment more 'ASD-friendly'?

How can you work with other members of the school team to make this happen?

Points to remember

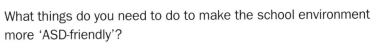

To ensure a stress free environment, consider:

- Whole-school issues
- Classroom issues
- Sensory issues
- Individual preferences
- Health and safety

3

Inclusive practice and whole-school approaches

This chapter examines the process of inclusion and the factors that need consideration if schools are to meet the needs of all pupils, including those with ASD.

Inclusive schools

In order for school to be fully inclusive they may need to review their current policy and practice with a view to change. The *Good Practice Guidance* (DfES, 2002) can be used as a self-assessment tool for both schools and local authorities. For example, factors such as:

- Clear channels of communication between agencies
- Support for parents during assessment
- Targeted training for professional groups like GPs, health visitors and playgroup leaders

are rightly highlighted in the Identification section of the *Guidance* (pp. 38–41).

Byers (1998) examines inclusive education within the framework of personal and social development and identifies the following factors for success:

- Ethos, spirit and atmosphere
- Rules, routines, rituals and respect
- Curriculum policy and schemes of work
- Meeting individual needs
- Teaching and learning

- Observation, recording, assessment and accreditation (see Chapter Six)
- Monitoring and evaluation

Given the social difficulties a pupil with ASD faces, it may be a useful model/measurement tool to adopt. The *ASD Good Practice Guidance* also provides schools with a useful and detailed checklist to evaluate the schools provision/inclusion of pupils with ASD.

Ethos, spirit and atmosphere

Byers (1998) suggests that in order for the ethos, spirit and atmosphere of a school to be conducive to inclusive practice, schools should examine their:

- commitment to equality of opportunity
- recognition and celebration of the value of the culturally, spiritually and socially diverse nature of society
- pupils' entitlement to an inclusive whole curriculum
- opportunites for all pupils to be involved in meaningful learning opportunities.

He argues that these factors should be explicit in the school's policy statements. Creating the right sort of ethos and atmosphere for pupils with ASD will not happen easily. A great deal of time will be needed to evaluate the school atmosphere and environment (see Chapter Two) and helping both pupils and staff to understand life from an ASD, rather than a neurotypical (NT) perspective. Changes will not take place without the commitment of the senior management team (SMT) and a dedicated group of teachers who are willing to learn more about ASD and cascade that information to others in the school.

Rules, routines, rituals and respect

Byers (1998) suggests that all pupils should be part of the decision-making processes in school. Pupils, including those with ASD, can be part of the process as members of the school or class council. Pupils with an individual education plan (IEP) should be encouraged to plan and monitor their own progress.

Funky Dragon (2002) have developed a participation checklist entitled 'Showing Respect'. It offers the following advice on pupil participation from the pupils' perspective:

- Involving us in deciding/organizing what/when/where
- Making sure adults don't take over the consultation
- Having fun – making the consultation more interesting

- Not making it too intense – user-friendly activities to facilitate change
- Paying attention and taking notes – don't talk, listen
- Liaising with decision-makers
- Finding ways to make us heard in public
- Letting us know what is going on
- Talking afterwards and explaining things

CASE STUDY

A young man with a fascination for newspapers and magazines was encouraged to make a newspaper-style portfolio to tell people about his strengths and needs. The point here was to produce a document that worked for the individual rather than impose the usual format.

(From The Handbook of Good Practice: Pupil Participation' (WAG , 2003a)

Curriculum policy and schemes of work

Byers (1998) posed the following pertinent questions for schools:

Does the school enable pupils and/or ex-pupils into certain curriculum development parties?
What is the appropriate balance between work addressing pupils' personal and social development and other aspects of the whole curriculum?
Do pupils have access to their full entitlement to whole curriculum concerns such as education and guidance about sexuality, spirituality, citizenship, morality, economic self-sufficiency or careers?
Are there options in the curriculum, particularly at Key Stage 4 and beyond? (pp. 56–7)

Although the National Curriculum has undergone changes and with creative and flexible thinking it can meet a diversity of needs, these questions can still be usefully employed as an audit tool and to encourage reflective practice.

Meeting individual needs

Most schools today are used to hearing the terms 'planning for differentiation' and 'responding to diversity'. IEPs are an obvious tool for meeting individual needs where a pupil is at School Action or School Action Plus of the Graduated Response (SEN Code of Practice). IEPs for pupils with ASD will inevitably target social communication, social interaction, flexibility of thought and developing independence. It could be argued therefore that the IEP is an effective instrument of inclusive practice. However, this will only be the case if it is set in the context of whole-school life and is not seen as something that is 'done' to the child away from the mainstream. IEPs are often seen as relating only to academic subjects but where the pupil's difficulties are social, IEPs can help to provide stategies and support at critical social times.

School staff will need to think about a range of groupings to extend and motivate learning on an individual basis. A range of activities may take place in the school day, e.g. whole-class teaching, paired work, pupil–other adult work, individual work or resource-led work. Each child in the school will have a preferred way of working. The pupil with ASD is likely to be happy with independent work (at their own workstation) and resource-led learning (ICT). However, this does not mean that they should not be encouraged to cooperate in other school activities such as whole class/group work. In such circumstances, school staff need to gauge stress levels and place a time limit on such an activity based on individual need and tolerance factors. Resources, worksheets in particular, in the classroom will also need to be evaluated in the context of individual need:

- Are they relevant to the pupil in terms of interest, ability and context?
- Is the resource intended for group work or individual work?
- Are language, layout, graphics, photographs appropriate? Do they distract from the meaning/are they misleading or ambiguous?
- Are they flexible enough to allow pupils to work at a different pace and a variety of levels?
- Do they allow for different learning preferences?
- Do they reinforce prior learning?
- Do they promote the transfer of knowledge and skills across the curriculum?

Other issues for consideration

In addition to their very specific needs, some pupils with ASD may have other issues that will also need consideration. They may have co-morbid conditions such as ADHD, dyslexia or dyspraxia or there may be particular ethnic/cultural/religious and language issues that will need to be given consideration in any teaching programme. When working with family members from local ethnic communities, jargon around ASD should be avoided and simple terms and examples used. Bear in mind that until only recently, in some community languages there has not been a word for autism (Dobson and Upadhyaya, 2002; Perepa, 2002).

CASE STUDY

Working together with ethnic minority communities

In 2000–2, a working partnership between two health agencies and a local autistic society undertook to research the experience of families from ethnic communities when receiving a diagnosis of ASD for their child. The partnership team felt that basic information about the triad delivered in the range of community languages most prevalent in Birmingham – Urdu, Punjabi, Gujerati, Cantonese, Bengali and Hindi – in leaflet format would help to further explain the triad.

The leaflets allowed parents to receive the diagnosis in a medium that they could access; the information could be shown to other family and community members as well as being mailed to wider family members who were not resident in the UK. Further information is available from www.autismwestmidlands.org.uk or via e-mail from l.a. plimley@bham.ac.uk

---

Teaching and learning

Adapting teaching styles to meet individual needs and motivate all pupils to learn is a key factor in inclusive practice. Teachers must bear in mind their own preferred learning style and consider a range of different ways to present information. For the pupil with ASD this will mean presentations that are visual, structured and use unambiguous language.

Monitoring and evaluation

Inclusive schools need to have efficient and effective systems of monitoring policy, practice and the progress of all pupils. According to ACCAC (2000):

> Evaluation is the process by which teachers make judgements against criteria/performance indicators to assess the effectiveness of actions on educational progress. The process needs to focus on the individual pupil to ascertain the most effective teaching/learning strategies as well as the effectiveness of the whole curriculum in the meeting of the needs of different groups of pupils in the school. (p. 28)

A range of people, with the support of the SMT and governing body, need to be proactive in this process.

Byers (1998) argues that monitoring and development should be used to drive forward developments in relation to:

- Ownership
- Social climate
- Policy, curriculum and schemes of work
- Revised IEPs and enriched teaching and learning
- Increased pupil participation and opportunities to contribute to the process through pupil interviews, diaries, and consultation
- The enhancement of learners' personal and social development.

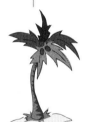

REFLECTIVE OASIS

How inclusive do you consider your school to be? Are there any systems in place to plan for, monitor and evaluate how inclusive your school is?

How do you make sure that your pupils with ASD are fully included in the life of the school?

Points to remember

- If inclusive practice is to work, everyone will need to be involved and a wide range of factors relating to school life will need to be explored
- Inclusion is a process and will need careful monitoring and evaluation

Planning the curriculum for access and accreditation

This chapter gives an overview of the curriculum at Key Stages 3 and 4 and Post 16. It examines both traditional and flexible approaches to access arrangements and accreditation.

Key Stage 3

For pupils aged 11–14, planning should start from the KS3 subject programmes of study. However, a high level of flexibility is provided through the access/inclusion statement which allows schools to use material from earlier (or later) key stages. For pupils with more complex needs, subjects may be used as contexts for learning and to address individual priorities, such as communication and social skills. There is now an increased emphasis on cross-curricular key skills including communication, personal and social skills and thinking/problem-solving. Although it will be necessary to 'take stock' of pupils' achievement during this key stage, the focus should be on assessment for learning which will provide information for teachers which informs their future planning.

Curriculum 14–19

The curriculum for young people aged 14–19 should be designed to secure equal opportunities and to offer a learning experience that will enable everyone to achieve their potential.

There is increasing emphasis on transferable key skills which are needed to succeed in a range activities in education, training, at work and in everyday life. Key skills are accredited at Levels 1 to 4 in the National Qualifications Framework (NQF; **www.qca.org.uk/493.html**) and defined as:

- Communication
- Application of number (AON)
- Information and communication technology (ICT)
- Problem-solving
- Improve own learning and performance (IOLP)
- Working with others.

For youngsters with ASD, the key skills could be addressed within the PSHE, citizenship and other social skills programmes, such as the Social Use of Language Programme (SULP; Rinaldi, 1993) and Circle Time (Gold, 1999), in addition to National Curriculum subjects.

It is important to include careers/work-related education, community participation and sporting/leisure and creative opportunities. These areas can be addressed in a number of ways to suit individual needs, settings, teaching and learning styles. Staff should gather information about pupils with ASD, including their views, and use this to inform planning. Pupils' learning styles (often visual), past experiences, and areas for development need to be considered in the development of a suitable individualized learning programme. Pupils should be encouraged to take responsibility for their own learning by setting targets, reviewing progress and recording achievements. Feedback on progress and certification for achievement should be given whenever possible.

Accreditation at Key Stage 4 and Post 16

The curriculum at Key Stage 4 and Post 16 should be based upon both present and future needs. For many pupils with ASD, it will be necessary to focus on independent social skills, work-related skills and leisure activities as well as National Curriculum requirements in order to ensure continuity between school and post-school life.

Achievement in National Curriculum subjects and personal and life skills can be accredited through the National Qualifications Framework which, in addition to GCSE/GCE, includes entry level awards for pupils working at a level equivalent to level 1, 2, or 3 of the National Curriculum. Details of approved general qualifications can be found at **www.dfes.gov.uk/selection 96/general/index.shtml**. There is also a range of vocational qualifications which may be appropriate for some pupils. Any programme of study will of course need to be based on individual needs and abilities and should still provide opportunities to address individual priorities.

In addition there are many opportunities for wider accreditation such as Duke of Edinburgh Award scheme, ASDAN, which may allow pupils with ASD to gain credit for their specific interests. Other credit award schemes such as AQA Units of Accreditation and Open College Network provide flexibility to accredit wider learning and also the learning of pupils working below level 1 of NC.

Useful websites are:

www.qca.org.uk/qualifications
www.accac.org.uk
www.qca,org.uk/openquals
www.ccea.org.uk
www.nfq.ie/nfq/en/TheFramework
www.scqf.org.uk
www.jcq.org.uk (Access Arrangements and Special Considerations)
www.patoss-dyslexia.org
www.nya.org.uk
www.batod.org.uk (Language of Examinations)
www.nocn.org.uk
www.aqa.org.uk
www.asdan.org.uk
www.dfes.gov.uk/curriculum_pre-entry/
www.dfes.gov.uk/readwriteplus/

Preparation for examinations

The Regulatory Authorities (Qualifications and Curriculum Authority [QCA], Qualifications, Curriculum and Assessment Authority for Wales [ACCAC], CEA [Ireland]) and Awarding Bodies are working to ensure that examinations are as accessible as possible to a wider range of individuals. Guidance for examiners (*Fair Access by Design*, 2005) will support the development of more inclusive GCSE/GCE examinations.

Loanes (1996) suggests that a range of strategies might be put in place to make life less stressful for pupils with ASD entering examination. These include:

- Providing a separate examination room
- Making a request for extra time
- Presenting the question paper on plain paper and in one colour
- Ensuring that instructions are clear, unambiguous and do not contain abstract ideas, except when an understanding of such ideas is part of the assessment

- Prompting the candidate when it is time to move on to the next question. (Such a request might be necessary due to an obsession with a particular topic and reluctance to move on).
- The use of word-processors or scribes when motor control is impaired.
- Requesting that the paper has been scrutinized by someone with a knowledge and understanding of ASD in terms of language and layout.

In oral tests Loanes argues that examiners will need to be made aware that candidates may:

- not understand body language
- try to get close to the examiner
- avoid eye contact
- make inappropriate remarks or noises
- echo questions
- have stilted speech unless the topic is a special interest, in which case it may be difficult to stop or divert a conversation
- fail to understand jokes, metaphors, exaggerations and take things literally
- not be able to respond to a question that relates to a social situation or involves the candidate looking at an issue from another's point of view.

It is important that, during KS3, teachers work with pupils and their parents to give early consideration to options to be taken at KS4. In addition, schools should make early contact with awarding bodies about possible access arrangements which may be available for examinations.

CASE STUDY

Access arrangements

At the end of Key Stage 3, the results of standardized tests, specialist support, past IEPs and any documents that relate to the history of provision are reviewed.

Using such information, the SENCo consults with pupils, parents, subject teachers and later the school examinations officer. S/he makes sure that access arrangements are put in place for tests and assessments at Key Stage 3.

(Continued)

(Continued)

Options at Key Stage 4 are considered.

Access arrangements for examination and qualification at Key Stage 4 are given early consideration.

Discussions take place with awarding bodies regarding any evidence required to ensure eligibility for access arrangements.
Pupils can access examinations as independently as possible (use of keyboards, etc.)

Where adjustments are to be made, the pupil is familiar with procedures.

REFLECTIVE OASIS

Consider a pupil with ASD in Year 7. How are you planning to meet his/her needs in terms of an appropriate curriculum and maximizing performance?

What issues do you need to consider for assessment in order that he/she shows true potential?

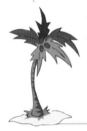

Where would you seek advice on ascertaining exactly what special arrangements a pupil with ASD might need to access GCSE examinations?

Points to remember

- Adopt a flexible approach to curriculum and accreditation
- Consider special arrangements well in advance
- Use interests for wider accreditation

Social strategies: helping pupils to cope

This chapter explores the problems that pupils with ASD might face in social situations at school. It gives examples of a range of published and unpublished strategies that might be used to reduce tensions.

Whitaker (2001) notes a range of problems that someone with ASD might face as a result of their problems with social communication and social interaction.

These include:

- Being frightened or stressed by contact with other people
- Being bothered about pleasing other people/making friends
- Causing offence without realizing/appearing insensitive
- Misunderstanding people's intentions
- Not knowing when to join in
- Going too far without realizing
- Not knowing how to react to other people's feelings
- Forming and keeping friendships
- Keeping a conversation going
- Knowing if another person is interested
- Being unable to read body language/tone of voice
- How tell if someone really means what they are saying (pp. 7–8)

Such difficulties can in some instances create big problems for your pupils with ASD. Nita Jackson (2002), a young woman with Asperger syndrome, explains how she feels:

Having taken an introspective view of myself, I am now able to see the cause behind me being socially inept, and if I was a mainstreamer I do not think I could tolerate the Asperger in me. I'm not the most endearing person – not because I'm defensive and nasty, but because of my desperation for friendship. I try too hard to make friends, and mainstreamers recognize this and can detect my insecurity (and consequently my inferiority complex). (p. 75)

Karen (cited in Sainsbury, 2000) also expresses her concerns about the social environment:

School was a torture ground in itself for me because of my lack of social skills and my absolute terror of people (in part because I didn't just automatically know the social rule, and, when I did learn them, I had to think about them all the time – and who can keep up that sort of coping skill ALL THE TIME). (p. 71)

Bullying

It is appropriate at this juncture to raise the issue of bullying and individuals with ASD. Social skills differences can lead to vulnerability. If one is looking for peer group approval and friendship, being different in the adolescent years is not a good thing. Many individuals with ASD recall the torture of being bullied at school and will say that very often they did not complain because they did not realize that they could. Maybe they had been told that 'Bullying is when someone keeps hitting you. If this happens you must tell the teacher.' But what if they were not being hit instead, they were being pushed and called names? To them this would not be a definition of bullying and something therefore they just had to accept.

Sainsbury (2000) highlights the magnitude of the problem with two examples:

I got hanged (with wire around the neck) and other kinds of what the staff called mild teasing ... no-one helped me ... things for me were somewhat more than the teasing issues ... it was torture and abuse.

I was bullied a lot because of being odd or different and they knew they could do it to me without me fighting back or reporting it to a member of staff.

Luke Jackson a young man with Asperger Syndrome, offers some advice to teachers. He says that teachers:

- should always be prepared to listen and take pupils seriously
- be discreet and not announce in the class that someone is being bullied
- should not tell pupils with ASD that 'they bring it on themselves'
- should not wander around the yard looking for bullying but rather sneak into locker rooms or dark corners of the school
- take the issue seriously and make it stop.

Social stories

Advocated by Carol Gray (**www.TheGrayCenter.org**), social stories can be used to help pupils with ASD to learn how to handle certain situations. Gray suggests that certain types of sentences should be used in the story:

> *Descriptive:* To define what happens – where, why and what statements. Occasionally it may be useful to use the word 'sometimes' to give flexibility.
> *Directive:* To state the desired response in a given situation and phrased in positive terms. It is better here to use terms like 'will try' rather than 'will do'.
> *Perspective:* To describe the behaviours, e.g. feelings, reactions, responses, of others involved in the situation.

Gray says that ideally the story should include two to five descriptive and perspective statements for every directive statement to ensure that it does not become a list of instructions.

Social stories involve interaction with and reinforcement by others. They must be consistently applied so that if inappropriate behaviour does occur they can be used to cue into appropriate behaviour.

When writing a social story for older children, involve them in the process. Decide together upon the behaviour that is causing problems and where it is most likely to occur. It may be necessary to involve other people in order to give consistency. It is important to ascertain that the perceptions of the story are fully understood by the pupil and that it contains small steps to ensure success. For some pupils it may be necessary to illustrate the story with drawings and photographs. The story will need to be used on a regular basis and monitored carefully to gauge whether it has brought about a change in behaviour.

Social sentences

The theory behind social stories has been used to create 'social sentences' for use with some youngsters with ASD. Social sentences can be used to help those with ASD to make sense of certain social situations. For example:

- Sometimes people don't answer when you talk to them
- Maybe they did not hear you
- Maybe they weren't paying attention
- Maybe they were busy
- I can forget about it, maybe they will answer me later

Social skills groups

In many areas social skills groups have been established in order for individuals with ASD to come together and learn about appropriate social behaviour. Nita Jackson (2002) discusses the social skills group she attended and says how valuable she found it to be. Her group was set up by Essex Social Services and consisted of seven young people with Asperger Syndrome and four teachers. Nita describes the teachers as friendly and open-minded who encouraged the group express themselves. She states that they never said a harsh word or used raised voices and this had a very positive effect on everyone.

Some social groups, like the one Nita attended, are highly structured and follow a special programme. Each session may focus on a specific issue, e.g. personal space, interrupting, bullying, making choices, interpreting feelings, predicting and avoiding danger. Other groups, however, might have been established simply to allow youngsters with ASD to get out and about socially and engage in a range of leisure activities. Some schools are now recognizing this need and establishing after-school clubs and Saturday clubs for pupils with ASD. When organizing leisure activities, it may be necessary to undertake a risk assessment.

Circle of friends

A circle of friends has the purpose of assisting young people with disabilities to adapt to settings (Whitaker *et al.,* 1998). A circle usually consists of six to eight volunteers who meet on a regular basis with the 'focus child' and an adult. The circle has three main functions:

- to offer encouragement and recognize success
- to identify difficulties, set targets and devise strategies for achieving targets
- to help put these ideas into practice.

In setting up a circle of friends it will be necessary to gain support and agreement from the 'focus child' and parents, meet with the whole class to recruit volunteers, gain agreement from the parents of the volunteers and organize weekly meetings of the circle.

Some teachers might argue that this is too contrived a way of developing friendships and support. Where youngsters with ASD are in resource bases in secondary schools, they may choose to make their own circle of friends with 'like-minded' youngsters.

Social Use of Language Programme (SULP)

SULP (Rinaldi, 1993) aims to increase functional language by focusing on pragmatics. Learning about pragmatics helps pupils with ASD to:

- understand the meaning in conversation
- use features of interaction such as facial and non-verbal communication
- develop conversational structures
- examine the wider influence of communication – social situations, backgrounds, attitudes etc.

The SULP programme makes use of strong visual and graphic stimuli and deals with age-appropriate issues and everyday situations. It provides opportunities to practise new skills and concepts via motivating activities and fun tasks. It uses a multi-sensory and metacognitive approach to develop understanding as well as skills.

> **CASE STUDY**
>
> A youth group which includes individuals with Asperger Syndrome has activities that are highly structured and chosen by group members themselves. Each week the group plans the activities for the following week. Workshop sessions are held on such topics as club rules, friendship and relationships.

Other strategies that may help at school include:

- Anticipating problems in advance – looking for triggers
- Planning for break and lunchtimes
- Providing a safe haven and looking out for any evidence of bullying
- Providing simple rules for social conduct in school and in the classroom, taking care not to be ambiguous, e.g. 'Put your hand up when you want to answer a question' must be followed by 'then wait for a teacher to call your name to answer'
- Teaching that pauses are natural breaks in a conversation and may be a cue to come in but not monopolize
- Making tapes of a pupil's voice and discussing expression and feelings
- Using school CCTV footage to promote discussion on social/anti-social behaviours
- Encouraging friendships and 'buddy systems'
- Encouraging participation in after-school clubs, especially where a special interest is involved, e.g. chess, ICT, sport
- Organizing structured paired work during lessons
- Drama, circle time and role play
- Activities that help individuals to understand the meanings behind facial expressions using photographs, videos, circle time and role play
- Helping the individual with ASD to express feelings, especially at times when they may feel they are about to lose control, e.g. providing coloured cards that can be placed face-upright on the desk where green signals calmness, yellow feeling anxious and red signifies the need for some time out/calming down
- Using favourite soap operas, DVDs and comic cartoons to examine a full range of social situations and relationships. In the context of school, it may be useful to examine school-based drama such as the TV series 'Grange Hill'.
- Using a special interest to assist in socializing, e.g. chess tournaments, computer club, judo, etc.
- Holding ASD awareness sessions for staff and pupils, explaining how they can help
- Making sure that adult support can be available at break/social times as these can be critical times of stress.

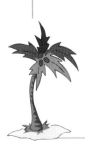

REFLECTIVE OASIS

How might you organize ASD awareness-raising sessions for other pupils?

Is there an opportunity for you to set up a social skills group/ circle of friends group after school or during lunch time?

How do you ensure that pupils with ASD are protected from bullying?

Points to remember

- Recognize that some social situations can be extremely stressful for pupils with ASD
- A wide range of published strategies can help
- Raise awareness of the issues across the school
- Give special consideration to break-times and lunch-times and those situations where bullying is likely to occur

Observation and recording

This chapter invites the reader to consider appropriate methods of observation for pupils with ASD and offers suggestions on purposeful approaches to assessment and recording.

Developing observational skills

When thinking about the child with ASD and planning to support them in the best way possible, it is always a useful exercise to spend some of your initial time observing the child in your setting. This may involve organizing tasks for the whole class to do independently and then taking short 5-minute bursts with a structured observation sheet to note down how the child is responding and what they are doing. It can also be useful to organize your class so that a support worker can do the directing, in order to free you up to do the observing.

Observation is a conscious process of systematized watching (Tilstone, 1998). We all do it in a variety of situations and settings, sometimes with a purpose, but often without a particular focus. Some of us are good at it and others may not pay sufficient attention to detail to glean useful information. We assume that we are doing it all the time, including in our professional lives. We can cite instances where our observational skills have put forward an hypothesis which has later proved to be correct.

> **CASE STUDY**
>
> Sarah, a teacher, noticed that Bea, a girl in her class, had a set of particular behaviours before she had a major epileptic fit. Currently Bea's condition was not stable and consequently she was experiencing

(Continued)

many absences during a school day and at least one major *grand mal*, where she would drop to the floor. Before the longer absences (around 10–15 seconds) and definitely before a *grand mal*, Bea would suddenly get out of her chair and go over to disrupt the work of her classmates. She would also ignore pleas for her to take her seat again and generally became 'stroppy'. Her out-of-seat behaviour increased the risk of Bea hurting herself if she had a *grand mal*, particularly if she was over by another child's desk.

Sarah developed her hypothesis about a behaviour onset of epilepsy over time and in order to prove the connection, she asked the support worker to make a focused record of these instances.

After compiling records for a week, Sarah found that her 'hunch' had been correct and she and the support worker were able to devise a plan of action in order to minimize the risk of Bea hurting herself. The record also proved invaluable to the consultant involved with Bea's condition and to her parents and family.

REFLECTIVE OASIS

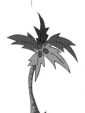

Have you ever noticed something that you later found to be a fact?

Is it important to write down medical details; who would benefit from it?

What are the consequences of not passing on this type of information?

As teachers, we feel we are automatically mentally recording many observations during the course of the day. What happens to our mental records? They often do not become a written record and sometimes they are not verbalized and disseminated at all. However, in teaching, the skills of observation and the data yielded are of critical importance to what we do and how we do it. Observation helps us to pinpoint needs, extend experiences and provide the building blocks for further learning.

Here are some ways in which we can use observational records to our advantage:

When observing the child with ASD, we can look at:

Behavioural changes in a child
How an individual interacts with different people
How the environment and different personnel can affect the child
How behaviours can alter according to the pressures of the circumstances

---

There are many such instances where observation can build upon hunches we hold or help clarify what governs a child's response. A variety of systems can help us to collect observational data. These could be observing:

- Individuals in a prescribed time period to record their interactions with others
- Individuals learning a new skill and collecting a record towards their success
- An individual's skills which are altered according to changes in staffing or the timetable
- Observing the child during an average school day to build up data on types of requests and activities they experience.

Before deciding on how to collect the data arising from these differing types of functions, you should ask yourself the following questions:

- What did the learner learn?
- How did the learner learn?
- Why did the learner learn?
- What appeared to get in the way of learning?

Although we may try to keep our observations as factual and objective as possible, there will be a subjective influence. To be completely objective we would have to operate in near-laboratory conditions, but we cannot replicate this in our classrooms. By formalizing the data collection, we can work towards being more objective.

Methods of observational recording

Video and audio

Video and audio can be a very illuminating way of observing. It can aid a more thorough analysis of particular aspects of classroom practice. The material you record will stand as a permanent objective record of what actually happened and it can be viewed or listened to again and again. Pivotal points can be explored and consequences can be investigated.

Advantages of videoing:

- It can be a permanent record and you can use it to view and review actions again and again
- The record can be used with others – parents and professionals – and be used to closely analyse particular features
- This type of record is helpful in looking at body language and non-verbal responses

Disadvantages of videoing:

- The position of the camera can give an incomplete picture of what is happening
- It can take a long time to find the actual piece of recording that you are most interested in
- The equipment may be difficult to obtain, set up and it needs checking that it is working (battery problems are quite common)
- The intrusion of a camera on a tripod or attached to a person may distract and disturb the objects of your observation

---

Tilstone (1998) argues that audio has an advantage over video because it can be made less intrusive.

Advantages of audio-taping:

- It can be a permanent record and you can use it to hear the recording again and again
- The record can be used to review specific points and check on particular details
- You can lend the tape to others for their feedback on the recording
- This type of record is helpful in following particular hypotheses that you want to check out

(Continued)

(Continued)

Disadvantages of audio-taping:

- Making recordings have the same drawbacks as video
- Playback and reviewing recordings can take a long time

Many classroom practitioners prefer to use methods that are seen as being more spontaneous and less reliant on cumbersome equipment and its inevitable maintenance. One such method is continuous recording. This requires a person to decide on a time slot or series of time slots during a specific subject/activity and to focus solely on child and a particular detail, e.g. communication; eye contact; possible behaviour triggers.

Advantages of continuous recording:

- The observer can get the breadth of what is happening and be able to keep a broad, objective picture
- The observer may be able to pick up on things that are unexpected
- This method can be used to give a series of titles/foci for a deeper period of observation
- It can be set up quickly and does not require too much forward planning

Disadvantages of continuous recording:

- In a busy room, the observer may be unable to record everything that a child says or does
- The observer may find something that they want to pursue and lose their specificity
- They may fail to notice some things and thereby their intended focus is lost
- They may have an ulterior motive (bias) and their recordings are not a true representation of what is happening

The final method is the use of 'nudge sheets'. Bailey (1991) believes they can be an effective '*aide-memoir*' to remind the observer about the specific factors that they are observing. Bailey says that a nudge sheet can set the context, and structure the observations in an effective but not too formal way. Here are some examples of how a nudge sheet can be used:

To focus on the contextual factors – where child is sitting, how available the equipment is, proximity of others
Physical circumstances – how child is sitting, height of table/desk, sensory issues
Task-related factors – how has the instruction been given, does child understand what is needed, what visual back-up is there for the task?
Communication issues – length of instruction, use of visual cues/schedule, child can ask for help

The teacher as a participant observer

Participant observation is likely to be the most frequently used way of observing pupils in the classroom by practitioners, be they teachers or support workers. If you can develop the ability to reflect on your own practice, then you develop opportunities for continuous review and improvement.

Cohen and Manion (1980) say that there are two main types of observation – participant and non-participant observation:

> In the former, the observer engages in the very activities he sets out to observe. Often, his 'cover' is so complete that as far as the other participants are concerned, he is simply one of the group … A non-participant observer, on the other hand, stands aloof from the group activities he is investigating and eschews group membership. (p. 101)

Cohen and Manion say that the non-participant observer can sit at the back of a classroom and classify the exchanges between teachers and pupils. A participant observer is a person who is involved in what they are observing. It can be argued that non-participant observers are better placed to gather systematic and objective data.

Points to remember

- Observe the pupil in a number of settings
- Some methods of observation can be less intrusive than others
- Make sure that assessment and recording have a purpose

Working with sensory differences

This chapter discusses the full range of sensory issues that might impact on learning and behaviour.

The work of people on the autism spectrum has contributed much to our insight into the experiences of people with the condition (Williams, 1992, 1996; Lawson, 2000; Grandin, 1995a, b). They report that all of their senses can at one time or another be affected by distortions and disturbances, making their experiences very different from ours.

Imagine that a child and his/her parents are looking for a suitable place for the next school move. Upon entering the new school there are noises coming from the rooms, raised voices, rapid and unpredictable movements of children/people in the corridors, staff calling out after children, ringing telephones and a loud buzzer signaling the end of the lesson. In your understanding of ASD, would you want to continue with the visit?

Common sensory differences

Here are some ways in which sensory differences may impinge upon the child in your school.

Visual

Visual distortions

The Channel 4 'A is for autism' video illustrates the ways in which people with ASD have reported that their sight can be blurred or distorted. Sometimes everything seems to taper down in dimension or things can look longer/bigger/smaller/shorter than they actually are. Most will say that this is not a perpetual way of perceiving the world, just that these distortions can happen from time to time and cause them deep anxiety. Others will find it hard to focus directly on things and prefer to use squinted eyes or the sight at the edge of their eyes – peripheral vision. All of these things combine to give some differing visual perceptions of situations. Dyslexia is a common condition for people with ASD and pupils you are working with may have been prescribed coloured filters – Irlen lenses (**www.irlen.com**) – to help them with their reading and organisation.

Useful strategies

Check different coloured filters (coloured 'paddles' are often used by science/art teachers). See if there is a particular preference that the child uses.

Watch their free play. Are they seeking out particular visual sensations?

If a child refuses to enter a setting, it may be because of a dislike of lighting/temperature or humidity.

Visual likes and dislikes

It is quite common for people with ASD to have some strong likes and dislikes in terms of patterns, colours and sequences. Their fondness for similarity may mean that they seek the visual experiences that make them feel secure. Always consider strong visual likes and dislikes and work towards extending and extending the experiences of the children you work with.

Useful strategies

Find ways of incorporating their patterning and colour sequences or repetitive drawings into a valued skill – make them the designer of a part of a display; use the patterns to create designs around the classroom – coloured containers for pens and pencils.

Show them that there is a value and an application of their work, but also that there are times when they have to do what is requested.

We all have our own visual preferences – symmetry, straight-hanging pictures, chairs and tables just so, for instance. If their preferences do not hinder, then do not try to change them.

Auditory

Hearing anomalies

A test of hearing is often one of the first medical interventions that parents seek for their child. Sometimes it appears that their attention is elsewhere but when you expect them to act upon your request they do so perfectly. Often they do not respond to loud repetitive sounds (heavy metal music for instance) but can become distressed by smaller, quieter noises that we do not notice at all (a person breathing too closely to them). These anomalies make us curious to find out exactly what they attend to and why. They may have a love of certain phrases or be able to memorize and reproduce a piece of video narration, including the tones and inflexions of speech that they would not normally use. A common sign of auditory overload is a child holding their fingers over their ears or partially covering the outer ear.

Many find music very relaxing and the use of personal stereos or iPods can be utilized effectively to override noise distress. It is also a highly effective and socially acceptable coping strategy.

Useful strategies

Forewarn of sudden noises – if you know there is going to be a fire practice, let the child know. Suggest some simple ways of either drowning out the noise (the iPod idea) or minimizing its disruption. Many secondary schools have used inventive ways of acclimatizing children with ASD to the end-of-lesson bell.

Where a child appears to having distortion in their hearing, imbalance in the ear or other aural conditions may be the cause of the distortion. Medical attention may be needed. If the child tells you that it only happens at certain times, then analyse why this could be. Could it be the acoustics in certain rooms or the tone/timbre of certain voices?

Tactile

Tactile defensiveness

This is an overreaction to any type of unwanted touch. Some report feeling assaulted by the touch of others. Others say that certain forms of touch are acceptable and others are not.

Useful strategies

Identify strong dislikes and introduce activities that contain elements of their defensiveness.

Replicate the ways in which close proximity may be needed in other activities – a simple 'trust' game of being blindfold and guided around by others may break down some of these defences.

If you work on identifying what type of touch they prefer (many prefer firmer holds, rather than stroking or gentle massage) and build up instances where that could be applied, then these defensive barriers may get broken down.

Tactile intolerance

Most of us cannot imagine how clothes and fabrics might hurt us, unless it's a too-tight pair of trousers, so we cannot know how certain clothing feels to the person with ASD.

Useful strategies

Materials like linen and cotton may be more comfortable and are easily available. Fastenings like Velcro and press studs may make it easier for the child with ASD to manage. Use information from home (parents will know best) to be guided by types of clothing and preferred fabrics.

Sometimes growing children approaching puberty will hang onto their familiar childhood clothes – this is because the fabrics may have softened and become more flexible with age. Working with parents may help to overcome difficulties when new clothing or sports items are bought.

Another reason to hang onto clothes they have grown out of is a fear of growing bigger and becoming an adult. This will need sensitive handling by school and parents to convey the appropriate information about body changes and growth spurts.

Olfactory and gustatory

Taste/smell predominance

People with ASD may have developed some strong preferences for food types, often focusing on foods with distinctive tastes (like Marmite and curries) or particular textures (crispy, smooth, chewy, crunchy). Within these preferences there may also exist some rigid rituals like only eating one food with another. Do not deprive them of their preferred food as you may find a child refusing to eat anything during school time. Show them that preferences will be catered for alongside the trying of something new. The pragmatic school will allow a child to bring their own lunchbox and not intervene with how that has been assembled.

You may come across someone who insists on tasting the new material put in front of them or smelling everything before complying with an instruction.

Providing the taste or smell is not going to upset them or, worse still, poison them, then this should be allowed. Once the new material or activity has been explored in this way, it is unlikely to need to be tasted or smelt again as it will part of the child's repertoire. If exploration by taste or smell may be dangerous, you have to respond in a way that the child knows means 'No, don't do that' or actively prohibit them doing so.

Useful strategies

Smell preferences could be noted and used as a relaxant, particularly if it is something generally soothing and calming to others, too.

For taste preferences, and restricted diets, then the advice is to persevere and take information from home. If a child is actively searching out food, then think about how to provide small amounts of food at regular times. It may not be greed, it may just be hunger or thirst, especially for pre-pubescent teenagers and those who are growing at a marked rate.

Other sensory considerations

We automatically think of the five senses when we consider the differing ways in which we process information. More recent work by occupational therapists (instigated by Ayres, 1979) and a psychiatrist (Hinder, 2004) would suggest that there are two other senses that help us in processing. Proprioception/proxemics and vestibular are both gross motor (whole-body) receptors.

Proprioception/proxemics refers to the way in which we position ourselves in space and time and know from infanthood how to keep a suitable distance from others. Vestibular is our innate sense of balance and knowing our capacities in exploring new experiences.

Proprioception/proxemics

Differences in proprioception/proxemics may affect the positioning of the body in space, the strength of grasp and the amount of awareness the person with ASD has of objects, furniture and people around them.

Although people with ASD have a very fixed, albeit invisible, boundary around themselves, they are no respecter of other people's personal space. You may not be allowed to approach them, but when they want something from you, you may find your space invaded. They may do that to any person that they perceive can fulfil a need for them and so this makes them particularly vulnerable when out in public.

The sense of personal space and when to apply different distances may need to be taught in meticulous detail – who is member of the public, who is a potential abuser, who is a member of my family?

Useful strategies

Work with them on recognizing the boundaries that they themselves apply and then transferring the same sort of consideration to others. Perhaps it would be better to teach the safe distance first and then work on letting favoured others come closer. Using the distance of an arm's length is a good guide.

If you encourage communication whenever, and wherever, then a quoit or a laminated coloured cross to mark where the child should stand can be thrown down on the floor as the communication begins.

Other ideas for the more able child might include using a social story (Gray, 2000) to illustrate what is close enough and too close. Using humour or rhymes will appeal to many children.

Vestibular

Children appear to lack fear of danger or falling, even when in the most precarious position. They may actually seek out these types of dangerous experiences.

What about children who love spinning, carrying on long after their peers would have collapsed in a nauseous heap? Or those who enjoy rocking, seesawing, hanging upside-down, swinging and fairground rides? These children with ASD are seeking out experiences that give them an extreme sensory 'high'. These can be used as a reward or to extend their knowledge of the outside world.

Useful strategies

Provide safe, acceptable alternatives in school. PE lessons give children the opportunity to scale reasonable heights and hang and swing upside-down.

Well-equipped schools have trampolining equipment – a great way of encouraging daring moves within a safe environment. For the child who loves climbing or running, athletics and outdoor pursuits are the way forward.

Climbing walls and outdoor centres are good choices. If you have risk – assessed the activity and have a qualified instructor, then the effects of being able to engage in such pursuits will teach the child the 'right time, right place' mantra.

Many special schools and ASD-specific schools have incorporated the principles of Daily Life Therapy (Kitahara, 1984) into their timetables and they use regular aerobic exercise as a means of preparing their children to settle down to work. The endorphins released by strenuous heart-racing exercise will also act as a de-stressor to the children (and adults) too.

Basic sensory approaches

- Many, but not all, people with ASD are visual learners and visual thinkers – think about how information is conveyed and expectations transmitted
- Incorporate visual timetables (Landrus and Mesibov, undated) into classroom and school practices
- Look at using ICT and multimedia to reinforce learning and skills; do not use teaching methods that rely on aural information
- Identify the sensory strengths of the child and work with those
- Discuss and initiate ways in which to build up the use and sensitivity of the 'weaker' senses
- Vary the sensory channel used in different activities – many school children will find this a challenge
- Think about the idea of 'monotropism' (Lawson, 2000; Williams, 1992, 1996) and focus on using one sense at a time
- Value the difference of experience that the child with ASD can offer to a class group. This should be respected and appreciated.

REFLECTIVE OASIS

Think about some of the children with ASD you are working or have worked with. List some of the ways in which they use their senses to gain information.

Make a list of how they spend their free time and whether this fulfils a sensory function for them.

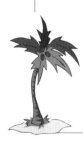

How could you use their sensory preferences to present new tasks?

What training opportunities would you identify for yourself and other staff?

Points to remember

- Consider the full range of sensory differences
- Examine the school environment in relation to sensory issues
- Use sensory preferences to maximize learning

Preparing for work experience and future employment

In planning for work experience placements and future employment, this chapter emphasises the importance making the most of skills for the future, forging links in the community and identifying roles and responsibilities.

The world of work: issues for consideration

It is usual for Year 11 pupils to have a one- or two-week work experience placement. Young people with ASD, like their peers, should be given the opportunity to experience the world of work. The experience of life in a work setting will give them an insight into good work habits and post-school aspirations. Work experience placements might also provide the opportunity to pursue a 'special' skill or interest. Surely, it would be a waste of resources if the skills acquired at school were not transferred to the workplace. Unfortunately, for many people with ASD this has not happened. But why? They have certain strengths that are ideal for the working environment. For example, they love detail and accuracy. They can retain their motivation and good performance on repetitive tasks better than most other people. They will never waste their time to engage in workplace chit-chat and gossip, or take long coffee breaks. They are honest, punctual, reliable and always stick to the rules. In addition, pupils with ASD learn best from real-life situations and access to work experience could equip them for life. Unfortunately, although these are all great attributes, one fundamental attribute is missing: the ability to communicate effectively.

More often than not, work and communication go hand in hand. At work, we often have to work as a team and we cannot overreact if a member of the team upsets us. There are certain protocols at work for how to relate to people. We get our jobs on the basis of an interview – a procedure which involves us selling ourselves using our communication skills. Often the work environment is not as comfortable as we might like. We may have to work in cramped office space, the lighting might be poor and the windows might rattle. We might experience changes in our working day – the telephone or an important email might interrupt what we are doing. Often we have to meet deadlines and therefore may need to compromise on the quality and standard of our work. Think about a young person you know with ASD. How easy would it be for him/her to cope with all these workplace situations?

CASE STUDY

A pupil in Year 10 with ASD who was due to start work experience was difficult to place because of inappropriate behaviour. As a result, it was decided that he should undertake his work experience placement within the school. He went to work in the school office, helped the caretaker and gave support to Year 7 pupils who found it hard to find their way around school. He was given a list of jobs to do on a daily basis and was guided by a member of staff. He kept on task and gained the respect of staff and pupils.

A group of teachers who attend Autism Cymru Secondary School Forum (2003) were asked what they consider to be key elements in preparation for employment. They suggested the following:

- Good preparation is crucial
- Prepare pupils in advance – find out what sort of job they might be interested in
- Research jobs on the Internet – what do you need to do to carry out certain jobs (interests, aptitudes, qualifications)?
- Look how to prepare – always being honest with the employer offering awareness training for staff if necessary
- Using visual schedules
- Teaching interview skills and the social rules of the workplace and the language of work
- Considering what will happen at break and lunch-times
- Identifying a work colleague who might act as a mentor
- Are there issues around medication?

These points might serve as a useful checklist prior to a work experience placement.

Planning the programme

Lee (2003) points out that transition from school to work can be particularly challenging for individuals with ASD because of their poor communication skills and social behaviour. He says that stress levels can be heightened by having to face new situations, routines, settings and meeting a range of staff. He warns that this might result in an individual with ASD becoming withdrawn and such behaviour could be misinterpreted as aloofness or rudeness by other members of staff who might then increasingly choose to ignore the individual.

The transition from education to employment therefore should be gradual and planned over a long period. This will include the young person with ASD having work experience prior to leaving school. Staff at school should liaise with the careers service as early as possible. The young person with ASD, their families and prospective employers must also be involved in the process. It will be necessary for employers to have awareness-raising in ASD. This could include the school making a short video emphasizing the positive attributes that an individual with ASD can bring to the workplace but alerting them to experiences in the workplace that may cause a person with ASD to feel stressed. It is important that employers are truly sympathetic.

Young people with ASD might find it difficult to cope alone in the work place. On occasions, they may need prompting because they do not understand the social cues. It is advisable for them to have a work-based mentor with a knowledge and understanding of ASD. The mentor could assist the young person with ASD with the work timetable and how to prioritize the day. A visual schedule would be useful in this respect. Strategies would need to be in place for dealing with highly stressful situations. A card system – or 'traffic-light' system (green for feeling good, amber indicating some stress and red indicating that the stress levels are becoming unbearable) could be used to alert the mentor that help is required. Facilities for a time away/calm-down period would need to be available in the workplace during such times. Lunchtimes and breaktimes in the workplace will need consideration.

Planning and preparation for employment need addressing in advance in the classroom as part of the curriculum. Social skills training for the workplace is vital if the placement is going to be a success. Marc Segar produced a very useful social guide for people with ASD. Segar emphasized that people with ASD need to be realistic about their choice of career. He suggested that suitable jobs might be graphic designer, computer programmer/technician/operator, research scientist and architect. He argued that these are respected professions which have colleagues who tend to be more accepting of the needs of those who worry. He said that people with ASD should avoid jobs that are highly stressful and may include making difficult decisions under pressure from other people, for instance, salesman, manager, solicitor, police officer, medical profession, teaching and airline pilot. Pupils should be encouraged to think positively about what they can realistically achieve and should collate a portfolio of evidence.

A personal portfolio can be particularly useful at interview and will emphasize the positives, since the young person with ASD is likely not to score highly in terms of communication, speaking and listening skills.

Lee (2003) describes work placement practices that have developed at a special school. Although the students in question will have had greater difficulties than many of their mainstream peers, the practice could form the basis of a model for either group. Lee refers to a 'work-related' curriculum. Work placements begin with a one day per week placement in the local community, e.g. shops, playgroups, hotels or homes for the elderly. For pupils with greater difficulties, 'in-house' placements can be arranged. Parents/carers are encouraged to become fully involved and their advice on a suitable type of placement sought. Lee emphasizes the importance of risk assessment for a placement. This will be crucial as many individuals with ASD may be unaware of heath and safety issues.

Students are provided with a gradual induction into the work experience placement. One student with ASD who becomes very anxious about change was provided with a social story to help him through this process. Students were kept on the same task for some period of time to help them get used to the changes in circumstances. Tasks were modelled for students and plenty of visual prompts such as photographs and schedules were provided. Lee notes that some potential employers were very nervous about participating in the programme. He argues that open communication and sharing of information are critical success factors.

CASE STUDY

A secondary school with a resource base for youngsters with ASD has developed a course known as Future Studies. The course aims to show pupils with ASD that everything has a purpose – school,

(Continued)

(Continued)

rules, parents, jobs, friends and life. It is designed to help individuals with respect to themselves and their future. It is learner-centred and encourages individuals to examine their own personal strengths and areas for development, what they perceive as opportunities and threats, their short- and long-term plans, and career opportunities and options.

Pupils are given detailed instruction on job applications, CVs, interviews, college courses, workplace routines and the role of the careers department, teachers and employers. They are prepared for their work experience by role play, preliminary visits to the proposed work placement and diary keeping. The school ensures that employers, pupils, carers and school work together to plan for the placement and consider what support might be required.

(With thanks to Janine Jerling)

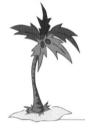

REFLECTIVE OASIS

What systems do you have in place to ensure that a work experience placement is successful?

Work experience should be a means to an end. What systems are in place to ensure that work experience and vocational training leads to employment in later life?

Points to remember

- Take time to plan and prepare for work experience with pupils and employers
- Accentuate the positives but recognize that the work environment relies on social and communication skills
- It may be necessary to provide support in the form of a mentor during a placement
- A work experience placement should be considered as a means to an end

Adolescence, sexuality and PSHE

> This chapter considers the difficulties that individuals may face as they reach puberty and adolescence. It examines ways in which the curriculum might address these issues.

Adolescence

Adolescence is a difficult period in most people's lives as they strive for their independence and try to detach themselves from childhood. However, for the young person with ASD it brings added difficulties and stress as they try to comprehend and cope with so many changes. Coping with change is not easy for individuals with ASD and like every other situation that involves change, planning and preparing for adolescence are crucial. Clare Sainsbury (2000) has Asperger syndrome and says that the most critical point in her life began in her teens. She states that very often individuals with ASD are 'late bloomers' and can reach their social and emotional 'adolescence' a decade or two later than their peer group. She argues that learning about social and sexual issues should therefore be ongoing and not time-limited. Sexuality is not static: it evolves throughout life.

Adolescence is a time when relationships with our peer group are most important. We want to be accepted by the group: we want to feel valued. The peer group supports our independence, meets our needs for identity, helps us develop the social skills and strategies for adulthood, provides us with entertainment, friendship and romance. Very often, individuals with ASD have not been accepted by their peer group as young children, so acceptance may be a problem in adolescence when idiosyncratic behaviour is tolerated even less.

Luke Jackson (2002), tells of how hard it is to stand out in a crowd when you so desperately want to blend in.

Adolescence is also a difficult time for many parents. Some young people move into adolescence creating few repercussions in the family, while others become rebellious in their search for independence. Parents of young people with ASD may see their son/daughter reacting in inappropriate ways to the physical changes in their body or they may have to deal with aggressive mood swings. It is yet another milestone which makes them reflect upon what is going to happen in the future and especially about the time when they will not be there to care. Schools must be particularly supportive of families at this time, helping them through the difficulties they may be facing.

CASE STUDY

The teacher in charge of a resource base for pupils with ASD in a secondary school has set up a parents' group. The parents meet one afternoon after school, while their children continue to take advantage of the school's ICT facilities. Although the teacher is present at the meetings, parents take the lead on the topics they wish to discuss. To date they have found it very useful to talk about a range of issues relating to personal hygiene and growing up – topics that are not always easy to discuss with others who are not experiencing such concerns.

(With thanks to Denise)

Developing a sex education programme

Moxon (2004) argues that for individuals with ASD sexuality encompasses the following key dimensions:

Moral

- Behaviours
- Religion
- Feeling
- Dilemma
- Attitude and beliefs of people in authority positions

Social

- Popular images
- Social opportunities

- Relationships
- The law
- The media, especially TV
- Communication

Biological

- Physical growth
- Development of sexual characteristics
- Being male or female
- Physical feelings including arousal
- Physiological responses to smell/touch/environment
- Genetics

Psychological

- Learned behaviours
- Self-image
- Gender and implications
- Attitudes around functions of the body
- Social cognition and perspectives

These dimensions can form the basis of an appropriate personal, social, sexual health programme for individuals with ASD. It important, however, to create such a programme in the context of individual needs. Often activities and tasks presented in a visual way or as a game can be used to highlight issues. Soaps and other TV programmes are also useful as a starting point for discussion or to scrutinize particular behaviours.

Wendy Lawson (2005) has Asperger syndrome and emphasizes the fact that the amount of support, advice and guidance given will depend on individual need. Different life experiences and intellectual capability will have an effect on the training programme required. She states that for many individuals with ASD, sex education will need to be learned in a highly structured way using concrete strategies. She recommends the use of pictures, photographs and videos, but warns us not to let the emotive components of sexuality cloud the overall objective. She argues that too little information and incomplete concepts can result in the person with ASD behaving in an embarrassing and unacceptable way. She cites the TEACCH programme (www.teacch.com) for sex education as a useful training example. There are four components to this programme:

- Discriminative learning (what to do, when and how)
- Personal hygiene (where, how often, changing underwear)
- Body parts and functions (sexual organs, male and female roles)
- Sex education (from friendship to sexual intimacy)

Based on this model , it is important for the key aspects in any teaching programme to include the following.

A focus on bodies, such as:

- naming of male and female sexual body parts using the correct biological terms
- discussing the differences and the similarities between males and females
- learning the facts about menstruation, erections, wet dreams and the menopause.

A focus on the physical and practical aspects of sexuality, such as:

- masturbation
- same-sex activity, including law, sexual health and consequences
- heterosexual activity, including law, sexual health and consequences
- contraception
- different kinds of sex.

A focus on the sexual/social aspects, such as:

- What does sex mean?
- Why do people have sexual relationships?
- How do we learn about sex?
- Who can/can't we have sex with and why?
- How can I keep myself safe?
- Is there a right time and a right place for sexual activity?

Other important aspects to teach, especially to individuals who are known to be sexually active, include:

- contraception and sexual health
- the importance of consent
- the consequences of sexual activity (physical, emotional and social)
- saying 'No' and coping with people saying 'No' to them

- what to do when sex feels bad
- the sexual rules that need to be obeyed.

A key point to remember in relation to any PSHE programme for individuals with ASD is their vulnerability for getting themselves into difficult situations. They need to be made fully aware of inappropriate touching and the dangers of invading personal boundaries. A lack of this knowledge could lead to them being accused of sexual harassment, or falling victim to sexual abuse/harassment themselves. For example, Jackson (2002) admits:

> I am always being told off for standing too close to people and following them around all the time but it is very difficult to know when it is right to follow someone around and carry on talking and when the conversation has ended and I am to leave them alone. (p. 164)

Such behaviour might be tolerated in a child but totally misconstrued in an adult. It is crucial that we make young people with ASD aware of this fact. Conversely, there is a risk of vulnerability of the individual with ASD to bullying and abuse from others. Some individuals with ASD can be over-trusting or may simply respond to the sexual stimulation without a clear understanding of the context. Programmes to help individuals with ASD to stay safe should make reference to:

- what to do if someone we don't know asks us to do something we are unsure about
- the difference between 'OK' and 'not OK' touching
- learning how to get away from an uncomfortable situation
- feeling safe – who can I trust?

Your approach to learning and teaching

Teaching a PSHE programme can be difficult because each of us has our own set of personal beliefs and code of moral conduct. We all have our boundaries. However, it is important to remain objective in this situation, helping individuals to make the right sorts of decisions without pressurizing them into our way of thinking and feeling. We may have to accept that people do not all think and behave in the same way. Everyone has the right to privacy and to express their sexuality in any way they want to, provided their behaviour is not hurting anyone else. Sometimes, there is also a danger of us projecting our own needs and thoughts onto individuals with ASD. For example, we may believe that individuals with ASD are incapable of having mutually satisfying relationships, irrespective of whether they want them. This view may permeate our teaching. There is a need therefore to set aside attitudes and remember that social interaction and developing relationships are a fundamental part of life and teaching related to this issue should therefore be a priority.

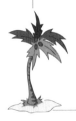

REFLECTIVE OASIS

How do you approach sex education for your pupils with ASD?

Are there any gaps in the content of your programme?

How do you check if concepts have been clearly understood in order to avoid inappropriate behaviour?

Points to remember

- Any PSHE programme must be based on individual need
- It must be structured and unambiguous and be taught in an objective unemotional way
- It will need to cover issues from personal hygiene to sexual intimacy

10

Developing partnerships with parents

This chapter focuses on the importance of working closely with parents and carers and ways in which information can be shared.

The Code of Practice

The Special Educational Needs Code of Practice in Wales and England emphasizes the importance of a genuine partnership between parents and professionals, especially during the assessment process. Many parents are not familiar with the 'graduated response' to assessment and feel concerned that without a statement of special educational need, their child will not get the services and help that they require. It is crucial therefore that parents are given as much information as possible. Under education law, it is important to remember that LEAs must make arrangements for parents to access Parent Partnership Services (PPS). It is important that parents are aware of the help and advice that PPS can provide. The Audit Commission (2002) says that most parents said that they had not found out about PPS until during statutory assessment, by which time their relationship with the school and LEA had often broken down.

The Audit Commission (2002) states that in most areas, parents complained about the information they had received about the assessment process; sometimes they were given too much information and had a difficulty in coming to terms with the jargon. The report also discussed the poor communication between professionals in different services and the insensitivity of some professionals as they worked their way through the system:

I'm fed up with the word 'professional'. It's like 'I am a professional and you are nothing'. But I am a professional on my child. They look down on parents... (p. 19)

Research by Wolfendale and Bryan (1994) recommends that:

- The school's SEN policy should be freely available to parents
- Information from the LEA, PPS and the voluntary sector should be displayed and made available to parents
- Home/school agreements should be used to promote parent partnership
- Schools should have a policy on parent partnership that includes details of contact and liaison issues with parents over SEN issues
- SENCos should have non-contact time to meet with parents and carers
- Schools should have clear lines of contact with relevant LEA personnel and voluntary organizations in order to increase their own awareness of SEN issues.

HM Inspectorate of Education in Scotland (2002) cite the following examples of good practice:

- Good home–school link arrangements to keep parents informed and involved in supporting their children's learning
- Steps to ensure that all parents can access communication from the school, for example, through translating newsletters into relevant languages and using plain English
- Partnership programmes for parents' own continued learning. Practical and accessible methods of making parents aware of what their child is learning and how they might help.

Disagreement resolution

The SEN and Disability Act (2001) placed a new requirement on LEAs to establish 'disagreement resolution services', an 'early and informal' means of resolving any disagreements with the LEA or school. This process brings together those in disagreement with a neutral representative. This service aims to prevent the long-term breakdown of relationships between home and the school/LEA. Accessing this service does not affect the rights of parents to appeal to the SEN and Disability Tribunal. The LEA and the PPS should be able to provide information on this service.

The SEN and Disability Tribunal

The Tribunal is an independent body which determines appeals by parents against LEA decisions on assessments and statements. From September 2002, the Tribunal was reconstituted to hear claims on unlawful discrimination on the basis of ability.

Parents can appeal to the tribunal if:

- the LEA declines to carry out a statutory assessment of their child following a parental request for assessment
- the LEA declines to make a statement for their child after an assessment has been carried out
- they disagree with Part 2, Part 3 or Part 4 of their child's statement when it was first made or later amended
- their child already has a statement, and the LEA declines to assess the child again or to change the name on the statement
- they disagree with the LEA's decision to cease to maintain the statement.

Meetings with parents

Parents of youngsters with ASD may become especially anxious when their child moves on to secondary education. Parents we have known have been concerned about the fact that their child might come into contact with a lot of other people who do not fully understand ASD and will react inappropriately. They worry also about incidents of bullying. School needs to be sensitive to these needs in any meetings that take place. Parents need to feel relaxed and confident enough to express their concerns to school staff. You must try to:

- be non-judgemental
- be sensitive
- be ready to listen
- be honest and specific
- be helpful
- avoid a 'them and us' situation by using clear language and ensuring that the physical layout of the room is welcoming and not threatening.

Parents are not having an 'interview' at school, but a 'meeting' with a view to working in partnership with school.

More formal meetings with parents like reviews or preparation of the IEP may involve the school in parental support prior to the event. This may take the form of a telephone conversation to discuss the agenda for the meeting or by giving the parents written details of the sorts of questions that will be raised. Some parents may feel more confident if they know in advance what they are likely to be asked and who is likely to be at the meeting.

During the formal meeting, parents should be given the opportunity to comment throughout. Clear and jargon-free explanations should be given. At the end of the meeting, action points should be summarized and agreed. Parents should be given a copy of the action points as soon as possible after the meeting. If a laptop has been used to take minutes, parents could have a copy of the action points immediately.

Fostering good home–school links

Any written information to parents should be user-friendly and as positive as possible. For the pupils with ASD who may separate home life from school life, home–school diaries can be a good way of maintaining communication between pupil, parents and school. They can also alert parents and school to any potential difficulties.

Some parents only associate telephone calls with bad news. Telephone calls also can be far more personal than the written word. When there is something positive or simply as a means of reassurance to a parent during those first few months in the secondary school, a telephone call noted on record can be a better way of making contact and encouraging partnership.

When youngsters travel to school in taxis or buses, parents can often feel very isolated. They may have a number of concerns as their son/daughter reaches adolescence. For some parents whose son/daughter has Asperger syndrome, a diagnosis might be fairly recent. Many local areas have parent support groups and it may be useful to inform parents about such groups or set up your own parent support group in school.

CASE STUDY

SNAP, Cymru's parent partnership service, offers a School Link Volunteer Scheme. School Link volunteers take general enquiries, disseminate general information, support the work of the SENCo, organize parent information sessions, encourage parent-to-parent contact, signpost support to other agencies and involve the wider community in the life of the school.

Transition planning (see also Chapter One)

First impressions are important, so it is vital that both parent and pupil are introduced to the school at least a term before admission. Parents should be provided with succinct and relevant information and be given the opportunity to discuss any anxieties. A video recording of life at the school could be particularly helpful to pupil and parent. Similar mechanisms will need to be considered when a pupil is to move on from school and should be in place by Year 9.

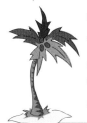

REFLECTIVE OASIS

How do you work with parents to ensure effective transition planning? Review the information you give to parents at this time. Is it succinct and jargon-free?

What systems are in place to monitor and evaluate partnership with parents in your school?

Consider your contact with parents over the last few weeks. What is your preferred method of communication? Are there any ways in which you could improve communication?

Points to remember

- Schools have a legal obligation to work with parents/carers
- Communication must operate on a number of levels
- Parents should be given a range of information from the school and the LEA
- Parents should be involved in planning for change or transition

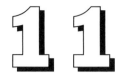

Managing challenging behaviour

This chapter considers ways in which stressful situations might be avoided and gives examples of the strategies that can be used to help pupils with challenging behaviour.

Avoiding stress and examining the triggers

The term 'challenging behaviour' is part of our everyday speech as an acceptable description of aggression, violence, and destructive behaviours. It is also a subtle adjustment away from the view that such behaviours are the responsibility of their 'owner' and emphasizes more the transactional view of the actions being a challenge to us to do something about. Work and theory around challenging behaviours (Zarkowska and Clements, 1994; Whitaker, 2001) put the responsibility on practitioners to analyse the reasons for the behaviour and devise a means of defusing its effects. We talk about inappropriate/unacceptable/harmful actions and sometimes even the word 'violence' is mentioned, but these labels are our own. For the person acting in a 'challenging' way the function of the behaviour might be to secure an escape or to calm them down. Repeated actions of this nature are often a way for them to regain control over a situation by producing a predictable set of responses from us.

We use the term 'challenging' because the behaviour being exhibited is not within what we would consider to be an acceptable range of responses. Extreme and repetitive challenging behaviours which have a definite sequence and from which the person finds it hard to move on become 'ritualistic', in our terms, and are viewed by us as imperative to control or extinguish. We feel the need to instigate an action/intervention to 'deal with the behaviour' but we often act in isolation and therefore inconsistent approaches arise. The key to effectively intervening in any response that we wish to shape or alter is to work together with important people in the person's life and the person themselves if possible, to teach more socially acceptable alternatives, including being able to articulate the cause of their discomfort.

CASE STUDY

John does not like going into assembly: he finds the room too large, too light, too noisy and the proximity of his peers too much to bear. John knows which days assembly is held. In the past John has shouted out, hummed loudly or rocked back and forth when he is in assembly. This has led to his form tutor removing him from assembly to go back to the form room. John disliked leaving the assembly because it meant having to negotiate his way through the legs and feet of his peers and their attempts to trip him up. Sometimes they also touched him as he passed. Although he was removed, it was uncomfortable and unpleasant for him.

John has developed a way of getting out of assembly before it starts. If he punches, spits or lashes out at his peers during registration, his teacher sends his class mates off to assembly and he gets to stay in the form room doing word searches with his teacher. His teacher is also less stressed because it has not been a public disruption.

This set of consequences has a predictable response for John and he has used his intelligence to think about how to avoid an unpleasant situation. He has refined his behaviours over time to minimize the fuss and discomfort of being removed from assembly. What he has never articulated however is the reason why he does not want to go into assembly. It would be a good starting point for us to begin to find the communicative function of John's behaviours.

Interventions that punish

Current belief is that seeking to punish or extinguish the unwanted behaviours of people with ASD simply does not work. Behaviourist theory of the 1960–70s advised intervention in the behaviour and introduction of a consequence that had an aversive effect (shouting, removal, physical punishment). Practitioners working in care and school environments would have been expected to find a way of stopping the behaviour recurring. Those working in those times may also have used corporal punishment, which had not then been legislated against.

A popular mistake of practitioners is to work to extinguish (remove) behaviour without giving a thought to teaching a more acceptable replacement activity. To punish and/or use aversive practices to respond to the behaviour will only teach the person anxiety/fear and a sense of discomfort. The outcome may be an element of conformity, but the person will not have a 'replacement' that gives out the same communication as the original behaviour. When looking at the practice of others, we see a group of children *conforming* and draw the conclusion that they do not have any challenging behaviours. We view conformity as a positive quality, indicating that everything is calm and learning is taking place. Not so with children with ASD. Conformity can be a learned behaviour – if being quiet, looking at the teacher and sitting still is valued, the child with ASD may do that in order to avoid further stress. It is a mistake to think that they are attending and learning at the same time.

Another popular technique in the 1970–80s was to ignore the behaviour. This could amount to negligence and result in personal harm if the nature of the behaviour was self-stimulatory. We have to think of the safety and well-being of the other children in our care and do our best to protect them from unnecessary harm. Current strategies/interventions carefully examine and interpret the function of the behaviour for the person. By looking at the underlying 'message', we are moving towards finding an acceptable replacement for it.

CASE STUDY

Ivan, a 12-year-old boy with Asperger syndrome, attends a mainstream secondary base for students with ASD. He joined the school midway through Year 8, having recently moved into the district. His referral papers documented a 'history' of volatile and unpredictable behaviour in his previous school.

The school's SENCo expressed misgivings, but the staff in the base were prepared to consider him, as they were well resourced and trained to meet his needs. They made a home visit and discovered that Ivan was talkative, friendly and good-humoured, keen to get back into school and learn. He was a sociable boy who would actively seek other peers to talk to and play with, although on his own terms and with little reciprocal interaction.

(Continued)

To help Ivan's transition, the school decided that attendance should initially be part-time and gradually increased over several months. A period of careful observation was undertaken and the teacher-in-charge worked with Ivan's parents to build up information and agree strategies. A weekly meeting, as well as the home/school diary and phone calls as necessary, were agreed. Subject staff were informed via briefing notes and suggestions for teaching students with ASD. During Ivan's first weeks at the school he was clearly stimulated by the academic demands of the classroom, but immediately presented staff in the base with challenges to their understanding and strategic planning. Some of Ivan's difficulties were quite similar to the other pupils in the base:

- Poor awareness of basic social rules and expectations, e.g. raising his hand to speak rather than shouting out
- He needed an occupation at breaktimes and lunchtimes as he had little idea of what to do
- His attempts to join in with others, consisting of pulling his chair closer and closer
- Occasional lashing out at other pupils gave some staff a feeling of nervousness
- Main-school teaching staff held the view of his behaviours as deliberate, targeted and intentional and attention-seeking

One lunchtime, Ivan threatened a member of staff. He spat in her face and twisted her arm behind her back. He was restrained by several people including a deputy head and a door was broken in this process. Ivan's father was called and Ivan was formally excluded for three days. The result of this incident was to devise a formal Pastoral Support Plan and a meeting prior to re-admittance allowed everyone concerned to reflect more closely on the behaviour and its causes. An analysis of the incidents of inappropriate behaviours over the 4–5 weeks revealed that at break and lunchtimes, Ivan could suddenly and unpredictably push or kick other students and staff. When he was removed from the room he offered no resistance and in discussion would admit that his actions had been inappropriate, although he was unable to explain it.

(Continued)

(Continued)

Ivan's father challenged the staff assumption that Ivan was attention-seeking. He thought that the behaviour was an expression of anxiety. He reminded the staff that the school was an entirely new environment for Ivan and that staff had probably assumed that because Ivan was articulate and had a sociable manner, he must also be confident and relaxed.

The incidents of challenging behaviour had occurred when there was lack of clear 'structure' and the expectation was that he could occupy himself.

Following this meeting a strategy was put in place to structure times out of class:

- A member of staff would spend time each morning with Ivan choosing from a menu of activities for breaktime (e.g. reading, computer, talking to a named member of staff/student)
- This was recorded on a sheet for later reference
- An agreed sequence of events was negotiated, including time for snack/lunch.
- A social story (Gray, 2000) was constructed around ways in which to join in with group activities if he wanted to
- A form of feedback, consisting of checking off the sequence of events on the prepared sheet, helped Ivan to self-monitor
- Each break/lunchtime that passed calmly without disruptive incident was marked with a star on another chart
- Four consecutive stars resulted in access to his MP3 player for the fifth day's breaktimes (Ivan had identified this as a motivating reward)

This simple approach was effective in substantially reducing the occurrence of the unwanted behaviour.

(Adapted from an original case study written for the webautism course, by kind permission of Olga Bogdashina)

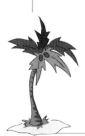
Points to remember

- Take time to observe pupils and record your findings
- Look for triggers and consider the issue from the perspective of your pupil
- Behaviour is a means of communication – so look for the message!

12

Issues relating to mental health and the criminal justice system

This chapter gives an overview of Mental Health services and the Criminal Justice system and the ways in which both might impact on the lives of individuals with ASD.

Mental health issues

During their lifetime individuals with ASD may come into contact with Child and Adolescent Mental Health Services (CAMHS). Indeed, an initial referral to the CAHMS team may eventually lead to diagnosis. Attwood (1998) notes that there are many sources of stress for individuals with ASD and their reactions can range from feelings of depression and anxiety to outbursts of anger and rage. Segar (1997) in his survival guide states that people with ASD are very good at worrying. He offers them advice such as 'talk to the right people not the wrong ones'. He suggests that 'right' people are teachers, relatives and sometimes friends. Using Segar's strategies for coping could help youngsters in your school.

Attwood explains that as a teenagers, individuals with Asperger Syndrome may become more aware of their social isolation and try to become more sociable. Their attempts to belong might fail, leaving them feeling excluded and depressed. Attwood argues that many young adults with ASD report extreme feelings of anxiety which can lead to panic attacks. He also makes the point that there will be a significant number of people diagnosed as having treatment-resistant or atypical chronic mental illness, especially schizophrenia, who will eventually be diagnosed as having Asperger Syndrome.

DfES (2001c) advise that schools can help to support the emotional well-being and learning of pupils with ASD by:

- having clear communication systems to ensure that children are clear what they have to do, where, with whom, when, for how long , what next and how
- ensuring that children with ASD have access to ways of learning that are appropriate for them, e.g. one-to-one teaching and instruction through a social means such as computer-assisted learning
- developing pro-social learning within the school to enable pupils with ASD to communicate and interact with others
- developing peer support systems, e.g. buddy systems and circle of friends (Whitaker *et al.*, 1998) in order to help those with ASD to manage free times and learn strategies to deal with potential bullying
- using counselling-type approaches to help pupils with ASD to understand misinterpretations of events/statements in the past.

Schools can also help further by:

- using discussion groups to raise a range of issues relating to feelings, emotions and anxieties
- recognizing the signs of stress before things get out of control, e.g. rocking, hand-flapping or other behaviours which are new or different
- providing equipment that might relieve stress such as soft balls, something to 'twiddle' with
- using social stories and comic strip cartoons (Gray, 2000)
- providing a safe haven (a room or place for relaxation)
- using relaxation exercises and physical activity
- providing stress and anger management sessions
- giving plenty of reassurance
- working closely with CAMHS to understand individual mental health needs much better.

CASE STUDY

Josh was diagnosed with ASD around the start of secondary school, and for the first two years he felt supported and happy. During Year 9, he began to be bullied by a group of older children, who tended to call him names and push him around in the corridors. The bullying carried on for a considerable time, despite intervention from the school to stop this. During this time, his attendance at school

(Continued)

(Continued)

became erratic. He began to leave school during the day when the bullying became too much for him. His mother noticed an upsurge in aggression towards her and his sister. When he got angry he also tended to break property in the house. On occasions, he stayed away from home and the police were called to find him. During this time, he did not speak to anyone about how he could no longer cope with this situation, despite other clear clues for others to pick up on. He became so despairing of any change happening at school that he attempted to hang himself in his home. Fortunately, he was found by his step-father, who was able to quickly seek help. Following this incident, he was referred to the local CAMHS team, and offered therapeutic support. These meetings in CAMHS were to address his self-esteem as well as problem-solve some of the social situations he struggled with daily. Within school, the SENCo spoke with the bullies and arranged a meeting for them with Josh. At the meeting, the bullies apologized and reassured him that the bullying would stop. This helped him because he was happy to accept that their apology was genuine. In addition, the SENCo offered regular meetings to encourage him to speak about any worries or difficulties before they might get out of hand.

REFLECTIVE OASIS

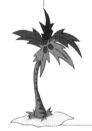

Think of a pupil with ASD who you work with. What are the possible triggers that alert you that he/she is feeling under stress/is likely to have an aggressive outburst?

How do you usually respond to the triggers? How successful do you think you are in recognizing the triggers and alleviating stress?

What systems are in place for close liaison with your local CAMHS team?

The criminal justice system

Sometimes young people with ASD may come into contact with the criminal justice system (CJS). The nature of their social difficulties, their trusting nature, certain 'special interests' and sensory sensitivity can make them particularly vulnerable in this context. Anti-social behaviour may occur because the social demands of others might cause them anxiety and lead to aggressive behaviour. They may:

- behave in socially inappropriate ways
- cause offence without being aware that they are doing so
- appear aloof, rude, egocentric and insensitive
- not know how to react to certain unknown situations and other people's feelings
- have difficulty understanding and using non-verbal communication
- not like to be touched in any way
- may have an extreme intolerance to certain sounds and smells or other sensory stimuli
- take things literally
- not be able to understand implied meaning or follow a long set of verbal instructions

Sometimes people with ASD can be the victims of crime; or because of a lack of awareness of heath and safety issues, they may be involved in an accident. In this event, they may become very anxious and react in a threatening and aggressive way. Their anxiety might be exacerbated by the change in their situation, a fear of the unknown and the sounds of sirens and being arrested. They can also react very differently to pain and could be in great pain without showing this.

What can you do to help?

Young people with ASD need to be prepared for any contact they may have with the CJS. Some voluntary organizations have worked in partnership with the police to produce a card for people to carry explaining their condition, as illustrated on page 74. It alerts the police and emergency services that ASD is a disability and individuals with ASD have the right of access to an appropriate adult or intermediary.

In the school context, the use of social-skills training programmes and social stories can help. It is also very important to involve your local Youth Offending Team and the Schools' Police Liaison Officer in any teaching programme. Those with ASD respond very well to rules and in this context it could be argued that they are less likely to get into trouble than most. Temple Grandin (1995a) argues that often people with ASD do

Tel: 01970 625256
www.autismcymru.org

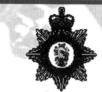

ATTENTION

I have an Autism Spectrum Disorder

* ASD is a disability
* I may need access to an intermediary
* Please ask questions one at a time
* Please tell me step by step what is to happen

North Wales Police

THANK YOU

Ffôn: 01970 625256
www.autismcymru.org

Autism Cymru

CYMERWCH SYLW

Mae gen i Anhwylder Sbectrwm Awtistaidd

* Mae ASA yn anabledd
* Efallai bydd arnaf angen help gan rywun
* Plis a wnewch chi ofyn cwestiynau un ar y tro
* A wnewch chi ddweud wrthyf gam wrth gam
  beth fydd yn digwydd

Heddlu Gogledd
Cymru

DIOLCH

'bad' things because they are not taught the rules. She has divided rules as follows:

Really bad things (murder, stealing, arson)
Courtesy rules (queuing, table manners)
Illegal but not bad (speeding, illegal parking)
Sins of the system (sexual misbehaviour, taking drugs)

CASE STUDY

A young man with ASD who witnessed petty theft in a shop was asked by police officers, 'Were you involved in the incident?' His response was 'Yes' and he was arrested. It took police officers some time to discover that the young man's interpretation of the word 'involved' was quite different from theirs. To him being 'involved' meant being at the scene of the crime rather than committing it.

REFLECTIVE OASIS

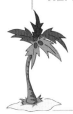

Consider the 'triad of impairment' and the implication that this might have in terms of involvement with the criminal justice system. Based on your thoughts, what systems can you realistically put in place in schools to act as a preventative measure?

Points to remember

- Feelings of social isolation can lead to mental health problems
- Stress levels must be kept to a minimum
- Social impairment may lead to an involvement with the criminal justice system as a victim or an offender, so teaching for prevention needs consideration

13

Educating colleagues

This chapter offers suggestions on raising whole school awareness of ASD and assists the reader in planning a presentation or INSET for colleagues.

Raising staff awareness

When including children with ASD into your mainstream school, it is important to make sure that everyone on the school staff has a basic awareness of the condition. This is true of other conditions too, but the differences that manifest in the child with ASD may baffle your colleagues. They may feel de-skilled and demoralized because the usual strategies in managing a class have failed. It is quite common to request someone from a local support group or ASD charity to address the whole school staff or there may the expectation that you, in your role supporting the inclusion of the child, will run a training session on ASD.

When you are preparing a talk or presentation to colleagues with whom you work, you may feel nervous and apprehensive. You may be concerned about the content of your presentation. Ready-made INSET materials are available (Hanbury, 2005). What you say could have an impact on school practice and so whether you use your own material or take comfort in someone else's, your commitment to and enthusiasm for the issues must ensue.

Conversely, speaking to a group of people who you will never see again can also raise anxieties. However, your style may be more factual and objective because you have not shared the same experiences or information. Both situations may necessitate that you admit to your own feelings and try to find ways of making the training experience as comfortable as possible.

Here is a checklist for a successful presentation.

- Is it appropriate and relevant?
- Does it convey respect?
- Is it objective and factual?
- Is it succinct and to the point?
- Is it delivered in an accessible medium – and one you feel comfortable with?
- Does it impart information that is important?
- Does it take into account and value everyone's point of view?
- Is it rooted in real life?
- Does it encourage the audience to reflect?
- Does it act as a catalyst for change?

When thinking about your audience, try to find answers to the following questions:

- Where are you giving this talk ?
- Is the location comfortable; will it have enough seating?
- Is the setting formal, e.g. a child/adult focus meeting, a team meeting? OR
- Is it informal, e.g. a lunchtime chat, a shift handover, a group of interested people/friends?
- How do you make sure everyone arrives on time?
- How long do you wait for people who are late?
- If people are late, how are you going to respond so that the atmosphere is kept light and accepting?
- Are you going to give permission to your audience to contribute or do you want to talk to them and then answer questions?
- Are you preparing handouts?
- If so, when do you give out your handouts – before or after?
- What have you got to keep your stress levels low and keep your voice from drying? A glass of water is recommended!
- Does your audience know something about the person/subject you are talking about?
- If not, how much background do you need to prepare?
- Have you got all of your materials to hand?
- Have you got a contingency plan (what if the equipment you want does not work?)
- Prepare an opening and a closing sentence that you can deliver without too much concentration. You can use your presentation as a prompt/script, but it's not important to learn it verbatim.
- Are you going to ask for feedback, to evaluate the effectiveness of your presentation?

Finally …

- Good preparation can never be substituted
- Spend time on your plan beforehand
- Test it against the previous key features
- Know how to keep yourself calm
- Get to the venue with at least 20 minutes to spare to give time to get ready
- Accept that you will have to deal with people turning up late; equipment playing up; and the unexpected
- Keep your voice level, at a reasonable volume and at a gentle pace – rushed speakers make their audience feel tense
- Encourage questions and comments – don't be afraid to say 'I don't know'. Ask if anyone else can help answer that question
- Find respectful ways of indicating that you agree with your questioner: 'That's a good point …' and to respectfully disagree: 'I'm not sure that I agree', etc.
- Don't forget to thank everyone for listening
- Make sure you give yourself five minutes after the presentation to relax.

CASE STUDY

You can lead a horse to water …

A teacher running a specialist support centre for children with Asperger syndrome attending mainstream secondary school was asked to raise awareness of ASD in her school. The centre had been set up by the county with only her to run it. There were three pupils diagnosed with Asperger syndrome attending the school at the time, each with his own remarkable set of 'challenging' behaviours. By the time she arrived, the staff had coped for a year with Asperger-fuelled outbursts of frustration, tapping, fidgeting, refusals to 'look-me-in-the-eye', etc. The boys had survived too (just!). The teacher had to move quickly to establish the 'support' that she was entrusted to provide.

Her first task was to speak to parents and support staff to find out as much as information as she could. Being new to the school, she needed to be diplomatic and not start telling experienced teachers how to do their job. She devised a questionnaire asking them for help in getting to know the boys. What worked? What didn't? Did

(Continued)

(Continued)

they feel they knew enough about ASD? Most admitted that they did not know enough. She decided to organize INSET.

60-plus high school teachers came to an INSET session after school. The designated teacher approached the session from a teacher's point of view. She gave a brief reference to the Triad and Hans Asperger and then on went on to what, she believed, was important to them – who were these children, how are they affected by ASD and, most importantly, how will their ASD affect them in the classroom. She provided pen portraits of each individual based on information from parents, support staff and her own observations. She summed up what the difficulties were likely to be, what the strengths were and, crucially, a few strategies to try to help make it work. She pointed out that some of the qualities and teaching styles widely accepted as those of a 'good' teacher would not necessarily work with a child with ASD, but having to search for a solution did not mean they had failed in any way.

During her time at the school, she has discovered that any resistance from colleagues is mostly as a result of finding it difficult to treat the pupil with ASD differently from another child – particularly when there is a need to be flexible with sanctions for inappropriate behaviour.

(With thanks to Gilly Hickton, Llandrindod Wells High School, Llandrindod Wells, Powys)

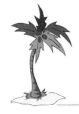

REFLECTIVE OASIS

Think about a speaker/lecture that has encouraged you to reflect upon your own practice. What qualities did the speaker have to motivate you? What resources were used to convey 'the message'?

Points to remember

- Think carefully about what you want to achieve – have clear objectives
- Think about your presentation in relation to the audience
- Comfortable surroundings are always appreciated

References

ACCAC (2000) *A Structure for Success: Guidance on National Curriculum and Autistic Spectrum Disorder*. Birmingham: ACCAC.

ACCAC (2003) *A Curriculum of Opportunity: Potential into performance. Meeting the needs of pupils who are more able and talented*. Birmingham: ACCAC.

Attwood, T (1998) *Asperger's Syndrome*. London: Routledge

Audit Commission (2002) *Statutory assessment and statements of SEN: in need of review*. London: Audit Commission

Audit Scotland/HMIe (2003) *Moving to mainstream*

Autism Cymru Secondary School Forum meetings 2003–5. **www.awares.org/edunet**

Ayres, A J (1979) *Sensory integration and the child*. Los Angeles: Western Psychological Services

Bailey, T (1991) Classroom observation: a powerful tool for teachers? *Support for learning*, 6(1), 32–6

Bishop, R (2001) Designing for special educational needs in mainstream schools, *Support for Learning*, 16(2), 56–63

Bowen, M (1996) 'Getting the balance right', pp15–20, in Coupe O'Kane, J and Goldbart, J (eds) *Whose Choice? Contentious issues for those working with people with learning difficulties*. London: David Fulton.

Byers, R (1998) 'Personal and social development for pupils with learning difficulties', in Tilstone, C, Florian, L. and Rose, R (eds) (2002/2000/1998) *Promoting inclusive practice*. London: Routledge, pp39–62

Channel 4 (1992) 'A is for Autism', available from **www.nas.org**

Cohen, L and Manion, L (1980) *Research methods in education*. London: Croom Helm

Cook, L L and Stowe, S (2003) Talk given on Nottinghamshire Inclusion Support Service at Distance Education (ASD) weekend. School of Education, University of Birmingham

DfES (2001a) *SEN Toolkit*. Nottingham: DfES

DfES (2001b) *Promoting children's mental health within early years and school settings*. Nottingham: DfES

DfES (2001c) *Inclusive schooling: children with special educational needs* (DfES 0774/2001)

DfES (2002a) *Autistic Spectrum Disorders. Good Practice Guidance*, Nottingham: DfES.

DfES (2002b) *Revised SEN Code of Practice.* **www.teachernet.gov.uk/teachingineng-land/detail.cfm?id=390**

Dobson, S and Upadhyaya, S (2002) Concepts of autism in Asian communities in Bradford, UK. *Good Autism Practice Journal*, October, 3(2), 43–51.

Fair Access by Design, (ACCAC): www.accac.org.uk/uploads/documents/2104.doc

Funky Dragon (2002) Personal communication to Maggie Bowen

Gold, D (1999) Friendship, leisure and support: The purposes of 'Circles of Friends' of young people, *Journal of Leisurability,* (26) 3

Grandin,T (1995a) 'How people with autism think', in Schopler, E and Mesibov, G B (eds) *Learning and cognition in autism*. New York: Plenum Press

Grandin, T (1995b) *Thinking in pictures and other reports from my life with autism.* New York: Vintage

Gray, C (2000) *The new social story book: Illustrated edition.* Arlington, TX: Future Horizons. **www.TheGrayCenter.org**

Hanbury, M (2005) *Educating pupils with autistic spectrum disorders.* London: Paul Chapman/Sage Publications

Her Majesty's Inspectorate of Education (Scotland) (2003) *Count us in*

Hinder, S (2004) Lecture on sensory differences in people with ASD. *Good Autism Practice Journal* Conference, Harrogate

Jackson, L (2002) *Freaks, Geeks and Asperger Syndrome.* London: Jessica Kingsley

Jackson, N (2002) *Standing down falling up. Asperger syndrome from the inside out.* Bristol: Lucky Duck Publishing

Kitahara, K (1984) *Daily life therapy. method of educating autistic children.* Boston: Nimrod Press

Landrus, R and Mesibov, B (undated) Structured teaching **www.teacch.com**

Lawson, W (2000) *Life behind glass.* London: Jessica Kingsley

Lawson, W. (2005) *Sex, sexuality and the autistic spectrum.* London: Jessica Kingsley

Lee, C (2003) Creating a work experience programme for students with autism, *Good Autism Practice Journal*, 4(2), 37–41

Loanes, J (1996) Autism and Asperger syndrome: Implications for examinations, *Skill Journal,* 56, 21–4.

Mesibov, G, Shea, V and Schopler, E (2004) *The TEACCH approach to autistic spectrum disorders*. New York: Plenum Press

Moxon, L (2004) Lecture on sex and sexuality with people with ASD. *Good Autism Practice Journal* Conference, Harrogate

National Qualifications Framework (2004) **www.qca.org.uk/493.html**

Perepa, P (2002) Issues in accessing support for families with a child with an ASD from the Indian sub-continent living in the UK. *Good Autism Practice Journal,* October, 3(2), 52–72.

Plimley, L (2004) Analysis of a student task to create an autism-friendly living environment. *Good Autism Practice Journal*, 5(2), 35–41

QCA/ACCAC/CEA (2005) Fair access by design

Rinaldi, W. (1993) *The social use of language programme.* Windsor: NFER

Sainsbury, C (2000) *Martian in the playground.* Bristol: Lucky Duck Publications

Segar, M (1997) *Coping: Survival guide for people with Asperger syndrome* **www.autismandcomputing.org.uk/marc2.htm**

Tilstone, C, Florian, L and Rose, R (eds) (2002/2000/1998) *Promoting inclusive practice.* London: Routledge

Tilstone, T (1998) *Observing, teaching and learning. Principles and practice.* London: David Fulton

Visser, J (2001) Aspects of physical provision for pupils with emotional and behavioural needs, *Support for Learning,* 16(2), 64–8

Welsh Assembly Government (WAG) (2001) *The SEN Code of Practice for Wales*

WAG (2003a) *'The Handbook of Good Practice'*

WAG (2003b) *Inclusive education (consultation document)*

Whitaker, P (2001) *Challenging behaviour and autism. Making sense – making progress.* London: National Autistic Society

Whitaker, P, Barratt, P, Joy, H, Potter, M and Thomas, G (1998) Children with autism and peer group support using 'Circles of Friends', *British Journal of Special Education,* 25, 60–4.

Williams, D (1992) *Nobody, nowhere.* New York: Time Books

Williams, D (1996) *Autism, an inside-out approach.* London: Jessica Kingsley

Wolfendale, S and Bryan, T (1994) *Managing behaviour; A practical framework for schools.* Stafford: NASEN

Zarkowska, E and Clements, J (1994) *Problem behaviour and people with severe learning difficulties.* London: Chapman & Hall.

Glossary

ADHD	Attention Deficit Hyperactivity Disorder
Aetiology	the root cause of a condition or disease
ACCAC	Qualifications, Curriculum and Assessment Authority for Wales
AS	Asperger syndrome
Autism Cymru	Wales' national charity for ASD
CAMHS	Child and Adolescent Mental Health Services
CJS	Criminal justice system
DfES	Department for Education and Skills (England)
DoH	Department of Health (England)
DSM IV	*Diagnostic and Statistical Manual* (Edition 4)
GAP	*Good Autism Practice* – a journal published by the British Institute of Learning Disabilities (BILD)
GCSE	General Certificate of Secondary Education
GCE	General Certificate in Education
HMI	Her Majesty's Inspectors of Schools
IEP	individual education programme
ICD 10	International Classification of Diseases

INSET	in-service training
LEA	local education authority
NAP-C	National Autism Plan for Children
NAS	National Autistic Society
NT	neurotypical
NVQ	National Vocational Qualification
NQF	National Qualification Framework
Ofsted	Office for Standards in Education: a non-ministerial government body in England responsible for the inspection of schools, LEAs, teacher-training institutions, youth work, colleges and early years provision
PECS	Picture Exchange Communication System
PHSE	personal, social and health education
PPS	Parent Partnership Services
SATs	Standardised Assessment Tasks
Secondary School Forum	developed by Autism Cymru to give teachers working with ASD in secondary schools across Wales the opportunity to meet and exchange information
SENCo	special educational needs co-ordinator
SENDA	The Special Educational Needs and Disability Act (2001)
SMT	senior management team
SNAP Cymru	The Special Needs Advisory Project in Wales
Social Stories	a strategy developed by Carol Gray to teach individuals with ASD appropriate social skills
SULP	Social Use of Language Programme
TA	teaching assistant
TEACCH	Treatment and Education of Autistic and related Communication handicapped Children
Triad of impairments	difficulties encountered by individuals with ASD in social understanding, social communication and rigidity of thought noted by Lorna Wing
WAG	Welsh Assembly Government

Index

Added to a page number 't' denotes a table.

access arrangements (case study) 25–6
accreditation, Key Stage 4 and Post 16 23–4
adolescence 53–4
anti-social behaviour 72–3
ASD Good Practice Guidance (DfES) 16, 17
Asperger syndrome 53, 54, 55, 70
atmosphere (school) 17
audio recording 36–8
auditory anomalies 41–2
Autism Cymru Secondary School Forum 49–50
autism-friendliness, in design 8
autistic spectrum disorders (ASD), social communication problems 27–8

behaviour *see* anti-social behaviour; challenging behaviour
bullying 28–9

careers, suitable 50–1
case studies
    access arrangements 25–6
    challenging behaviour 65, 66–8
    contact with police officers 75
    environment design 12–13
    mental health issues 71–2
    observational skills 34–5
    parents' group 54

case studies *cont.*
    respecting individual strengths 18
    School Link Volunteer Scheme 62
    staff awareness 78–9
    transition planning 3–5
    work experience 49, 51–2
    working with ethnic minority communities 20
    youth group 31
challenging behaviour, managing 64–9
    avoiding stress and examining triggers 64–5
    interventions that punish 65–6
Child and Adolescent Mental Health Services (CAMHS) 70
circle of friends 30–1
classroom design 10–12
classroom planning 9
co-morbid conditions 20
colleagues, educating 76–80
colour, decorating rooms 11
continuous recording 38
criminal justice system 72–3
curriculum 22–6
    accreditation at Key Stage 4 and Post 16, 23–4
    for ages 14–19, 22–3
    Key Stage 3, 22
    preparation for examinations 24–5

curriculum *cont.*
    work-related 51
    see also National Curriculum
curriculum policy 18

Daily Life Therapy 46
decision-making, pupil involvement 17–18
dedicated workstations 11
descriptive sentences 29
design, autism-friendliness 8
directive sentences 29
disagreement resolution services 60
dyslexia 41

education provision, types 2t
environment 7–15
    autism-friendliness in design 8
    classroom design 10–12
    classroom planning 9
    human qualities 10t
    new provision 8–9
    whole-school issues 7
    see also working environments
equipment 11
ethnic communities, working with (case study) 20
ethos (school) 17
evaluation 21
examinations, preparation for 24–5

Fair Access by Design 24
food preferences 43
furniture 11

Good Practice Guidance (DfES) 7
gustatory sense 43–4

hearing anomalies 41–2
home-school diaries 62
home-school links, fostering
    good 62
human qualities, working with
    ASD 10t

inclusion, pointers for
    successful 7
inclusive schools 16–21
Individual Education Plans
    (IEPs) 19
individual needs, meeting 19
individual preferences,
    consideration of 11
induction, work experience 51

key skills 23
Key Stage 3, 22
Key Stage 4, 23–4

learning styles 20
lighting 12

mainstream schools 2t
mental health issues 70–2
mentors, work-based 50
monitoring, policy, practice and
    progress 21

National Curriculum 18
needs, meeting individual 19
non-participant observation 39
nudge sheets 38–9

observation, participant 39
observational recording,
    methods 36–9
observational records, use of 35–6
observational skills,
    developing 34–5
olfactory sense 43–4
oral tests 25

Parent Partnership Services
    (PPS) 59
parents
    concerns, secondary
        provision 1
    partnerships with *see*
        partnerships
parent's group (case study) 54
participant observers 39

partnerships, with parents 59–63
    Code of Practice 59–60
    disagreement resolution 60
    fostering good home-school
        links 62
    meetings 61–2
    SEN and Disability
        Tribunal 60–1
    transition planning 62–3
Pastoral Support Plan (case
    study) 67
peer groups 53
personal portfolios 51
personal and social
    development 16–17
personal, social, sexual health
    programmes 55–7
    teaching 57–8
personal space 11
perspective sentences 29
planning *see* classroom planning;
    transition planning
portfolios, personal 51
pragmatics, learning about 31
primary schools
    education provision 2t
    transitions from 1–6
proprioception 44–5
proxemics 44–5
punishment, challenging
    behaviour 65–6
pupil participation, decision-
    making 17–18
pupils, helping to cope 27–33

recording *see* observational
    recording; observational
    records
respect, showing 17–18
ritualistic behaviour 64

schemes of work 18
School Link Volunteer Scheme 62
schools
    common differences
        between 2t
    inclusive 16–21
secondary schools 2t
sensory differences 40–7
    basic approaches 46
    common 40–4
    proprioception/proxemics 44–5
    vestibular 45–6
sentences, social stories 29, 30
sex education programmes 54–7
sexuality 54–5
smell predominance 43–4
social communication
    problems 27–8
social sentences 30

social skills groups 30
social skills training 50, 73
social stories 29–30, 73
social strategies 27–33
Social Use of Language Problem
    (SULP) 31
space (classroom) 10, 11
Special Educational Needs Code
    of Practice 59–60
special educational needs
    coordinators (SENCOs) 2
Special Educational Needs
    and Disability Act
    (2001) 60
Special Educational Needs and
    Disability Tribunal 60–1
special schools 2t
spirit (school) 17
staff awareness, raising 76–8
storage space 10
stress
    avoiding 64–5
    new situations 50
SULP *see* Social Use of
    Language Problem
support contracts 2

tactile defensiveness 42–3
tactile intolerance 43
taste/smell predominance 43–4
teachers, as participant
    observers 39
TEACCH 55
teaching styles 20
telephone calls, to parents 62
transferable skills 22–3
transition planning
    from education to
        employment 50–2
    from primary to secondary
        school 1–6
    partnerships with parents 62–3

vestibular sense 45–6
video recording 36–7
visual distortions 40–1
visual likes/dislikes 41
visual timetables 14

Webautism vi
whole-school issues 7
work experience, preparing
    for 48–52
    issues for consideration 48–50
    planning the programme 50–2
'work-related' curriculum 51
working environments,
    managing 14

youth group (case study) 31